WHAT AMERICA'S TOP DOCTORS ARE SAYING ABOUT JORGE CRUISE

"I'm eternally grateful to Jorge for creating a simple lifestyle plan."

—**Christiane Northrup, M.D.,**
#1 *New York Times* bestselling author of *The Wisdom of Menopause*

"Eat well without dieting or going to the gym with Jorge's strategies for breakfast, lunch, and dinner."

—**Mehmet Oz, M.D.,** host of *The Dr. Oz Show*

"Jorge Cruise gives practical advice for maintaining optimum health and weight by making food choices based on cutting-edge nutritional science. He explains why obesity is epidemic in our population and tells you how to avoid it and other health problems associated with the mainstream diet. Good information."

—**Andrew Weil, M.D.,** author of *Why Our Health Matters*

"Jorge knows, as I do, that excess sugar in our diets is among the most important factors conspiring against our waistlines and our health."

—**David Katz, M.D.,** director and cofounder, Yale University Prevention Research Center, and nutrition columnist, *O, The Oprah Magazine*

THE
100™

Also by Jorge Cruise

THE 100™

Count ONLY Sugar
Calories and Lose
Up to 18 Pounds
in 2 Weeks

JORGE CRUISE

wm

WILLIAM MORROW

An Imprint of HarperCollinsPublishers

This book is written as a source of information only. The information contained in this book should by no means be considered a substitute for the advice of a qualified medical professional, who should always be consulted before beginning any new diet, exercise, or other health program.

All efforts have been made to ensure the accuracy of the information contained in this book as of the date published. The author and the publisher expressly disclaim responsibility for any adverse effects arising from the use or application of the information contained herein.

THE 100™. Copyright © 2013 by JorgeCruise.com, Inc. All rights reserved. Printed in the United States of America. No part of this book may be used or reproduced in any manner whatsoever without written permission except in the case of brief quotations embodied in critical articles and reviews. For information address HarperCollins Publishers, 10 East 53rd Street, New York, NY 10022.

HarperCollins books may be purchased for educational, business, or sales promotional use. For information please write: Special Markets Department, HarperCollins Publishers, 10 East 53rd Street, New York, NY 10022.

FIRST EDITION

Designed by Jaime Putorti

Library of Congress Cataloging-in-Publication Data has been applied for.

ISBN 978-0-06-222707-2

13   14   15   16   17   DIX/RRD   10   9   8   7   6   5

To Lisa Sharkey:

Thank you for believing in my message, and for having the courage

and vision to illuminate the truth about weight loss, and giving

the world a real chance at ending the obesity epidemic. Your

support for this and our future books in *The 100*™ series will

continue to empower and inspire people around the world.

CONTENTS

··· P A R T   F O U R ···
Bonus Material

THE 100™

Foreword
by Dr. Vincent Pedre

When I was in medical school in the 1990s, very little time was devoted to nutrition. All learning was centered around which medications were best to treat particular conditions. It seemed that the only way to treat a disease was to reach for the script pad. But as I started my practice, I instinctively knew that something was missing in patient care.

My quest for more answers led me to become the "accidental" nutritionist. It was my patients' needs and their incessant requests for weight loss guidance that led me to want to study nutrition and weight loss science. I studied integrative and functional medicine to pursue my passion, and I realized that the best medicine was actually in the kitchen. The most powerful interventions I could inspire in a person were to lose weight and become physically active. In my practice, I help my patients understand the source of their weight gain, working on strategies to help them lose the weight by addressing the underlying issues.

Over the last several decades our understanding of the key role nutrition plays in our health has broadened immensely, but there are still many old ways of thinking we hold onto that are getting in the way of fully understanding weight loss. Looking at all calories as equal when it comes to weight gain is simply outdated science, yet many weight loss programs still pivot on the disproven concept of calories in = calories out. In *The 100™*, Jorge Cruise provides a clear, evidence-based explanation why the old way to count calories is not only wrong, it will certainly set you up for weight loss failure. *The 100™* offers a new way of counting calories, based on sound science. This new approach to weight loss is not only simpler and easier to follow, it will allow you to feel satisfied while watching the pounds effortlessly come off.

Simply stated, the problem that has been throwing a wrench in your weight loss efforts is insulin. After reading this book, you will understand how this ultra-important hormone plays a key part in weight gain, especially with our *carb-heavy* eating patterns. By making the connection between sugar, carbs, insulin and the accumulation of fat in the body, you will be empowered to make the right food choices. *The 100™* will change the way you think of which calories count and which don't. You will learn a new way to plan your successful weight loss and lifetime eating plan. This is not only a diet, it is a new eating mindset and lifestyle change.

The first time Jorge Cruise told me about his exciting new approach, we talked about the key role insulin plays in weight gain and many other diseases, such as prediabetes, diabetes, metabolic syndrome, cardiovascular disease, heart disease, and hypertension to name a few. High insulin levels are often missed by your doctor, who may only be doing a routine check for fasting blood sugar, which may be "normal" even if your insulin levels are high. Fasting blood sugar alone will often miss the mark. It is the ratio of your fasting blood sugar to your fasting insulin level that is more telling. A ratio greater than 7 should be your aim, keeping in mind that an ideal fasting blood glucose is between 70 and 90 mg/dL.

Further measurements, including BMI (body mass index) and waist circumference (a marker for insulin resistance) halfway between the belly button and the ribs—provide more information about unwanted weight gain. For women, a waist larger than 35 inches, and for men larger than 40 inches, is a sign of insulin resistance. If this is your waist size, your body has become insensitive to the signal insulin puts out—the signal that when recognized will move glucose into your cells for energy production, but when not recognized will lead to all of the diseases mentioned above. Ultimately, this is the main issue that has caused you to pack on the weight, and what is reversed by following the program in this book.

Knowledge is power. *The 100*™ will give you the right knowledge to conquer your weight for good. With a thorough review of the history behind diet science, and how we went astray after World War II with ill-advised diet plans, this book will walk you through a clear account of weight loss trends and why some worked and others failed. I always believe that the most important thing I can give a patient is knowledge and understanding of their condition, because with that they can find the right motivation to move forward. *The 100*™ will teach you what is going to work for your weight loss, and what won't. And this is based on more than 100 years of research from scientists and doctors around the world.

I have seen the enthusiasm with which Jorge Cruise motivates people like you to lose weight and stay fit. You will find that same level of enthusiasm and the right motivation through the words in this book. I have the utmost respect and admiration for his ultimate goal to make America and the world healthy. It starts right here with this new diet plan.

More than any time in history, we need to understand why our old way of eating is slowly making us sick and heavy. If only we can look at nutrition as our medicine, rather than waiting for the right pill to cure the disease, we will become empowered to make the right choices and live healthier and happier lives.

May you find inspiration in *The 100*™ to change your eating patterns, and ultimately to begin on your path to wellness.

Best wishes,
Vincent M. Pedre, MD

WELCOME

From the desk of Jorge Cruise

D ear Friend, get ready because I have some shocking news. Currently the US government suggests a Recommended Daily Allowance of 1,752 Sugar Calories or around 9 cups of sugar.

THE GOVERNMENTAL RECOMMENDED DAILY ALLOWANCE TRUTH

Note: when counting Sugar Calories we take into account ALL carbohydrates, since they are all sugar. With that in mind we see the following scenario play out:

- 10 oz carbohydrates = 130 carb grams = 520 Sugar Calories

- 2.5 cups fruit—Orange juice = 64 carb grams = 256 Sugar Calories

- 4 cups vegetables—Sweet Potato = 144 carb grams = 576 Sugar Calories

- 3 cups dairy—Skim milk = 36 carb grams = 156 Sugar Calories

- 2 servings added sugar—2 cups lemonade = 64 carb grams = 256 Sugar Calories = 1752

For years, experts, including government officials and health agencies, have been telling us that cutting overall calories is the key to weight loss, and that ending obesity is a simple matter of counting calories. *The 100*™ is perhaps the most breakthrough book on the subject of weight management to date, because it actually shows you where dietary science is today, and it is probably not what you are thinking.

I am thrilled to introduce to you The 100™—my easiest program yet. **If you cannot wait to see the newly updated science, I give you permission right now to find out the secret of this book located in chapter 3.**

Discover how specific foods cause your body to hold on to excess pounds and the simple changes you need to make to release excess fat from your body. The 100™ way of losing weight will keep you on the path to **lose up to 18 pounds in just two weeks!!**

So, if you're ready to see the truth about calories, and learn how you can eat all the delicious foods you don't want to give up then you are in the right place. Get ready for a smaller, more energized, vibrant you, now and forever.

I cannot wait to show you how it all works!

Your coach,

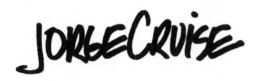

PREFACE

My Vision for You and for Our World

am incredibly blessed to have had the opportunities I do, and with these blessings has come great responsibility. That's why I've devoted my life to one critical mission: To spread the truth about obesity and being overweight with the hope that I can help as many people as possible to break free from the vicious cycle of dieting, temporary weight loss, and eventual weight gain.

I've experienced firsthand what it's like to struggle with weight. I was raised in a family where food was abundant and rich in refined carbs and sugars. Beginning at a young age I was taught to eat what was served to me, and to finish everything on my plate. Throughout my childhood and into high school I sought out sugary foods and refined carbs for comfort and to reduce the anxiety I felt, but also because, unbeknownst to me, these foods are also highly addictive. I didn't know they also fueled weight gain. It wasn't until I was more than 40 pounds overweight that I finally discovered the importance of the types of foods I was eating and what they were doing to my body and my health. Once I was able to understand that it wasn't that I was eating too many calories, it was the quality of the food, not the quantity that was the problem, I was able to change my way of eating, lose the weight, and stay healthy.

My goal is to change the way we view food on a global level, to change the way the whole world eats. That's why I've dedicated over a decade of my life to writing books, coaching men and women, and appearing on radio and television to spread my message—eating in a way that matches how the human body was meant to work is the key to ending our struggle with excess weight for good. I've done years and years of interviews with leading health experts, read hundreds of books as well as scientific studies on nutrition and weight loss, and I firmly believe that we've been led astray. The messages we've gotten over the years on how to lose weight have just been plain wrong—and I want to take you through my journey, because I believe that once you know what I know, you'll be as convinced as I am.

In my past work, I've focused on strategies that have people count and track the amounts of sugars and carbohydrates in food. This is still a good strategy, but I have evolved from my previous work to realize that the way the world thinks is in terms of calories. Calorie counting can, and has been, a hindrance in the past, and to some extent still is because when you count all calories equally you can easily overlook the essential and sometimes harmful components of a given food—specifically sugar. That's why I'm going to teach you *a new way of viewing calories.* The old view and the conventional wisdom—how much heat your food puts out or calorie counting—is out of date, and completely misleading. Not all calories are used equally. I know I'm treading on very controversial ground here, but the science is so compelling and life-changing that I want you to know every detail. That's what this book is all about.

Calories were invented to assist you in weight loss; however, the specific key to weight loss that works long term is to track only the calories that cause weight gain and fat storage. These Sugar Calories (see chapter 2 and chapter 3 to learn all about this culprit) have been hidden and misnamed by the food industry to such an extent that you've had no fair chance at losing weight successfully, despite your best efforts. That's about to change. I'm going to teach you a new way of doing the math that fits with how your body consumes and uses calories. Once you are informed, you'll never treat all calories as equals again.

We are in a global health crisis with ever-rising rates of obesity, diabetes, cancer, heart disease, and Alzheimer's, and my hope is that this book will teach you the common thread I see running through all these conditions—namely sugar, sugar, and more sugar. Armed with the knowledge in the following pages, you'll be ready to take control of your life and protect your health, and the health of those you love.

THE 100 | How to Use This Book

To simplify the wealth of material in this work, I've organized it for ease of use. This book is broken into four sections, and while you can feel free to jump ahead to the menus and food planners, I believe that you'll be more invested in The 100™, and will see better results, if you take the time to read this book in the order in which it is laid out.

In Part I, we're going to take a journey through the past to see how we got from being mainly healthy hunter-gatherers to the disease-burdened modern day people we are today. By taking this history lesson in chapter 1, you'll be able to see how the relatively recent changes to our diets have harmed our health, why scientists invented the "how hot your food gets relates to your weight loss" theory of calories and the hidden science that has proven correct. We'll also look at the introduction of refined sugars and grains, and the influential role of politics, personalities, and the food industry. In chapter 2, we will look at the science of what keeps human bodies healthy, what in our modern diets is harming our bodies, the specific role that carbohydrates and sugars play (Sugar Calories), and how to eat for health and well-being. We'll also look at what goes on in our bodies to cause chronic diseases, and how these are linked to carbohydrates and sugars as well.

In Part II, I'll teach you a new way of viewing calories. In chapter 3, you'll learn what Sugar Calories and Freebies are all about. By learning what calories are Freebies, and what calories should be tracked (Sugar Calories), you'll find a new freedom in eating and enjoying your diet, while being able to shed stubborn pounds. You will understand the components of various foods, how Sugar Calories cause weight gain, and you'll be introduced to new strategies of eating that match your genetic blueprint. Chapter 4 is where we take action with The 100™. You will learn about the menus and how you can lose up to 18 pounds in two weeks! This is a no-brainer food plan that I've made super simple—you won't have to track anything because I've taken care of the choices for you. The foods are all easy to find and prepare, so you'll enjoy four weeks of effortless eating.

In Part III, chapter 5, we'll look at how to move forward after you've finished your first four weeks on The 100™, how to eat when the going gets tough, and how to track and keep a food diary. Then, in chapter 6, get ready to get your motivation revved. Here I'll outline how to stay motivated no matter what challenge faces you.

In Part IV, chapter 7, I'll share specifics for how to add variety to your eating plan based on how you are feeling, and your special dietary needs. In chapter 8, you'll find extensive food lists for Freebie foods and Sugar Calories. In chapter 9 we'll take a look at how exercise works on The 100™.

Throughout the book, you'll see inspiring testimonials labeled "I Did It!" from clients who have found success using my philosophy for successful weight loss to keep you motivated. Also incorporated throughout the book are excerpts from an interview I conducted with my mentor, Gary Taubes, the award-winning science writer and author of Good Calories, Bad Calories, Why We Get Fat, *and* Bad Science. *Gary has opened the world's eyes to the issues surrounding obesity, not as an issue of calorie control, but as one of hormonal imbalance and food quality. He has helped me understand that the key to weight loss is found in understanding that not all calories count, and how insulin works in the body to control the regulation and storage of fat based on the types of calories you consume. He's inspired and informed much of my work and research, and now you can share in his words of wisdom by reading the boxes labeled* **Interviewing My Mentor.** *Since the interview excerpts are taken out of context, I've included commentary in italics when further explanation is necessary.*

I know that you can find a new freedom and a new happiness within the pages of this book, and I'm so excited to share it all with you. Let's get started.

PART ONE

The Foundation of Weight Loss

Even the most formidable building will turn to rubble without a solid foundation—the same can be said of successful weight loss. If you don't build your weight loss plan on what really works—your solid foundation—you won't be able to reach your goals. That's what these first two chapters are all about. I'm going to take you down memory lane to a time in history before humans knew of obesity. We'll follow these mostly healthy hunter-gatherers to the disease-burdened modern day people we are today. We'll also look at the introduction of refined sugars and grains, and the influential role of politics, personalities, and the food industry. In chapter 2, we will turn to the science to learn what in our modern diets is harming our bodies, and how to eat for health and well-being. We'll also look at what goes on in our bodies to cause chronic diseases, and how these are linked to carbohydrates and sugars as well.

The History of Heft

Those who don't know history are destined
to repeat it.

—EDMUND BURKE

The story of how we became a nation of more fat than thin individuals has its origins more than 10,000 years ago. Understanding how we went from then to now takes a bit of a history lesson, but it's a worthy use of your time, not to mention a fascinating story, because after reviewing the history of our growing plight you'll have an elevated insight into our hefty problems with obesity. Understanding how we got into this state of unhealth—from point A to B—is the first step to ending your struggle with weight forever.

You'll be rewarded with a new wisdom and a new freedom by taking the time to carefully digest this chapter, as well as chapter 2: The Science of Skinny. By the end of this chapter you'll understand how we evolved from healthy humans, virtually devoid of obesity—and most of its related diseases—to a culture dripping in fat. This new understanding is going to open your eyes to how you've been misled by public health officials and government agencies to repeatedly trust in flawed recommendations for losing weight—despite your most sincere efforts. With this new wisdom, you'll finally have the tools to shed the stubborn pounds and excess fat from your life forever.

Eating with Our Genetic Blueprint

Believe it or not there was a time in human history when being overweight and obese was a rarity. In fact, more than 99.5 percent of our genetic existence on this planet, some two and a half million years, was spent being mostly lean, healthy, and virtually disease free. This was known as the Paleolithic era or, less technically, the Stone Age, because it began with the development of the first stone tools. This accounts for more than a hundred thousand generations of living as hunter-gatherers, compared with just six hundred generations that we humans have been farming, or the mere ten generations of people who have lived in the industrial age (see "History of Eating Patterns" for a breakdown).

During our time as hunter-gatherers, we roamed the earth as tribes of peo-

HISTORY OF EATING PATTERNS

When you look at the human diet from a historical perspective, it's easy to see how our bodies evolved to eat food:

TIME PERIOD	DIETS	TIME FRAME	GENERATIONS OF DIET
Paleolithic Era, The Stone Age	Hunter-gatherers: high protein, high fat, leafy green vegetables, nuts, seeds, berries	2.5 million years	83,000 generations
Agricultural Era	Farmers: introduction of dairy, corn, rice, potatoes, and tree fruits	10,000 years	333 generations
Industrial Era	Introduction and dissemination of refined flours and sugars. Even more recent, the introduction of candy bars, chips, liquid sugars in juices, coffee drinks, teas, and sodas.	400 to 600 years	20 generations

ple who hunted and trapped small and large game, fished, foraged for seeds, nuts, vegetables, berries (the few months of the year they were in season), and, in smaller concentrations, for honey, eggs, and even insects. Experts believe that humans thrived as hunter-gatherer societies because we lived as animals in our natural habitat. British epidemiologist, Geoffrey Rose described this as "biological normality." In other words, this way of eating was under the conditions to which we were genetically adapted to consume food—we were eating how we were evolved to eat. Interestingly, obesity, being overweight, and the diseases of modern civilization (cancer, diabetes, Alzheimer's, and heart disease) do not appear to have existed until we started farming some 10,000 years ago, and then refining starches into flours and sugars (a mere two to three hundred years ago), which I'll address more fully in the next section. The former introduced starches such as potatoes and wheat as a regular part of the human diet, while the latter introduced processed foods completely devoid of nutrients. Each alteration radically increased the amounts of Sugar Calories consumed by humans.

The logical argument goes like this: Our agriculture period only accounts for 0.5 percent of our history as humans, and the time period for refining flours and sugars only covers 0.01 percent. When you compare this with the 99.5 percent of our past spent eating as hunter-gatherers, the food we eat today could be considered foreign, akin to giving soda to a lion.

The specific components of hunter-gatherer diets seem to have varied depending on the regions in which people were living. For example, in the colder or more drought-plagued areas, humans in the Stone Age probably ate high

Historical and anthropological studies show hunter-gatherers to be healthy, fit, and largely free of the degenerative cardiovascular diseases common in modern society.

—**James O'Keefe,** MD, preventive cardiologist best known for his studies in the field of cardiovascular medicine, professor of medicine at the University of Missouri–Kansas City, and coauthor of the bestselling consumer health book *The Forever Young Diet & Lifestyle.*

levels of proteins and animal fat, seeds, nuts, leafy green plants, some berries, starchy tubers, and honey when they could find it, while others ate higher levels of vegetables, seasonal fruit (most often berries), tubers, and lower quantities of meat. These eating habits are speculations to some extent because anthropologists were doing a majority of the detective work for a period before there was record keeping, but thankfully some modern-day hunter-gatherer societies still exist that can be used to extrapolate what was in our ancient diets (see "Ancestral Eating Habits" for more information).

In any case, what is most noticeable and assuredly true about all nomad bands of people is that high carbohydrate diets, refined carbohydrates, easily digestible sugars, high-fructose corn syrups, and sugar-laden foods and beverages that are so common to our modern-day lifestyles simply didn't exist. In fact, as Gary Taubes points out in *Why We Get Fat,* "many of these foods have been available for only the past few hundred years—the last thousandth of a percent of our two and a half million years on the planet." Even foods like corn and potatoes only became popular 500 years ago, while the mass production of sugars and flours has only been around since the 1850s. As historical researchers in a 2000 analysis put it: ". . . cereal grains, dairy products, beverages, oils and dressings, and sugar and candy comprise more than 60 percent of the total daily energy consumed by all people in the United States, these types of foods would have contributed virtually none of the energy in the typical hunter-gatherer diet." As you'll learn in the following pages, these foods are almost wholly comprised of Sugar Calories.

Interestingly, obesity, as well as the diseases common to Western civilization all follow the same trajectory throughout history, they increase dramatically with the addition of farmed grains and tubers, refined starches, and sugars. It boils down to this: As one rises—eating carbohydrates, refining grains, producing sugars—so do the others—obesity, diabetes, diseases. Considering all these facts makes it easy to see how straying from our ancestral eating habits has damaged our health.

ANCESTRAL EATING HABITS

Figuring out what our Stone Age predecessors ate is tricky business. While cave paintings do depict hunters with spears chasing down animals for food, our ancestors didn't exactly keep food diaries. Fortunately, some hunter-gatherer tribes did continue to exist far enough into the 1900s for anthropologists to assess their eating habits. The most comprehensive study of these types of societies was published in the *American Journal of Clinical Nutrition* in 2000. American and Australian researchers analyzed the eating habits of 229 hunter-gatherer populations that were still functioning into the 20th century. Here's what they found:

- Only 14 percent of the populations got more than half their calories from plant foods, and not a single group was vegetarian.

- When averaged all together, the researchers found that these societies consumed about 66 percent of their total calories from animal foods, and 33 percent from plant foods.

- Breaking it down further, the analysis showed that our ancestors ate up to 35 percent of their calories from protein, and up to 58 percent in fat calories, with some populations eating as much as 80 percent of their calories from fat (modern-day diets are around 15 percent protein, 33 percent fat, and more than 50 percent carbohydrates).

- The fattest parts of the animals were preferred in the Paleolithic era, according to the analysis—the opposite of the lean meats that are most popular today.

The carbohydrates that were part of the hunter-gatherer diet, while still a plentiful 20 to 40 percent, were high fiber and low carbohydrate seeds, nuts, roots, tubers, and leafy greens—all slow to raise blood sugar and slow to digest.

The Invention of Farming

As touched on earlier, our troubles with excess weight and other diseases first appeared with the birth of agriculture, and then, more recently, with the manufacturing of grains into flour, and cane into sugar. This began somewhere around 10,000 years ago. First, humans farmed in their natural native habitats by locating plants they liked and then protecting the plants from predators, which then progressed to tilling fields of grains and starchy vegetables we'd never find in the wild, such as corn, potatoes, wheat, and rice. This is how we initially began consuming far too many Sugar Calories than we are genetically designed for. It was with the introduction of these foods that our biologically natural diets were first displaced.

Scientists who study the historical effects of agriculture and nutrition report that these changes in eating habits are too recent on the evolutionary time line for our bodies to have genetically adjusted to the shift from protein and fat to carbohydrates. This displacement from a genetically friendly diet introduced too many Sugar Calories, which unnaturally increased the amount of insulin secretions in our body, and, as I'll get into in the next chapter; this spike in insulin caused our bodies to start storing more fat than we were using.

And farming was just the beginning. The most radical transformation of

The problem is when we take sugars and concentrate and refine them, and serve them in massive amounts throughout the food supply . . . That's causing hormonal changes that in many people drive hunger, cause overeating, and increase the risk of diabetes and heart disease.

—**Dr. David Ludwig,** a pediatric endocrinologist, director of the Optimal Weight for Life (OWL) Clinic, and the director of the New Balance Foundation Obesity Prevention Center at Boston Children's Hospital.

Today's panoply of diets—from fast-food burgers to various concepts of balanced diets and food groups—bears little resemblance, superficially or in actual nutritional constituents, to the diet *H. sapiens* and its ancestors consumed over millions of years.

—**Jack Challem,** columnist for the journal *Alternative & Complementary Therapies* and author of several books, including *No More Fatigue, Stop Prediabetes Now, The Food-Mood Solution, The Inflammation Syndrome, Feed Your Genes Right,* and *Syndrome X.*

our eating habits (until the introduction of high-fructose corn syrup in the late 1970s) was the refining of the cane plant and sugar beets into sugars and grains into nutritionally empty flour.

Radical Changes: Introducing Sugar and Flour

By the late 1700s, sugar and flour were common commodities across Europe, although both were primarily available to the rich because of cost. It wasn't until the mid-19th century with the invention of roller mills for grinding grain that flour and sugar became widely available. Shortly after, sugar beet cultivation spread throughout the civilized world. Both flour and sugar are made by removing (aka refining) all the fiber, nutrients, minerals, and vitamins from the whole grains and plants from which they come, and what you have left is a highly concentrated substance that is devoid of any essentials your body truly needs—in other words, they are non-essential (in the next chapter we'll get more deeply into the components of these foods and their effects on the body). However, sugar and white

"With flour and sugar came the introduction of jams, jellies, cakes, breads, and the addition of sugar to coffee and tea, and so on—and as these foods became more commonplace, so did obesity and diabetes."

flour were highly valued because they were seen as attractive to the eye, easily digestible, resistant to spoilage, and less liable to be subject to infestation by insects or rodents. They were handy, convenient, and long-lasting.

With flour and sugar came the introduction of jams, jellies, cakes, breads, and the addition of sugar to coffee and tea, and so on—and as these foods became more commonplace, so did obesity and diabetes, and with those came many cancers, heart disease, and other conditions.

As civilization spread across the world, nonperishable foods, such as sugars and flours and their resulting concoctions (biscuits, crackers, etc.), were shipped along as well. It was during this time, from the mid-1800s to the early 1900s, that many of the first reports of *diseases of civilization* or *Western diseases* such as obesity, diabetes, heart disease, high blood pressure, stroke, gallstones, and cancers surfaced. Most accounts from this time were written by missionary doctors who were on hand caring for hunter-gatherer populations when the transition to Westernized diets occurred. Physicians in North Africa at this time reported higher rates of cancer with "the advance of civilization," and by the early 1900s, doctors in Africa would rarely report cases of cancers in areas where natives kept their diets traditional, but these physicians detailed increasing rates of cancer in neighboring towns where "European" diets were incorporated.

This story would be repeated a multitude of times, with stories of populations that remained isolated from a Western diet exhibiting no disease or cancer, while in the United States rates of disease were on the rise, within the

What I'm saying is that our current food supply is so glutted with fructose, that is added sugar, sugar that was put there very specifically for the food industry's purposes, both for palatability and for shelf life, that it has now created a toxic—basically a toxic side effect in our livers, driving all of these chronic metabolic diseases.

—**Dr. Robert Lustig,** pediatric endocrinologist at the University of California, San Francisco, and star of the viral YouTube video *Sugar: The Bitter Truth.*

GARY: We know that there were populations that didn't have cancer. I mean it's documented in the literature from the 1870s onward. And you can follow it all the way into the present. In the Inuit Eskimos there was no cancer; the first documented case of cancer in an Inuit was in 1937. As late as 1967 you couldn't find breast cancer in Inuit women, but in American women one in nine women would die of breast cancer. And yet, it was a nonexistent disease among the Inuit. In Japan breast cancer is an extremely rare disease among Japanese women and when they move to the U.S. by the second generation they have the same breast cancer rates as anyone else.

[*The Inuit are the folks we commonly refer to as Eskimos—Inuit actually refers to a group of culturally similar indigenous peoples inhabiting the Arctic regions of Greenland, Canada, and the United States.*]

JORGE: Nothing has changed except the behavior—what they were eating?

GARY: When the researchers, the best epidemiologists in the world, look at these kinds of data and compare these populations to other populations and cancer rates (things like what happens when populations immigrate to another country), they concluded that as much as 70 percent of all cancers could be prevented.

As much as 70 percent could be prevented if we could figure out what foods, what aspects of lifestyle other than cigarettes were causing these cancers.

JORGE: And what are the foods?

GARY: Well, the obvious ones again are sugar and refined flours. But sugar, primarily.

JORGE: Sugar causes cancer?

GARY: You can argue and I can argue that sugar would be the prime suspect in most lifestyle-related cancers. The evidence suggests that sugar causes a condition called *insulin resistance*. When you are insulin resistant you have to secrete more insulin in response to the carbohydrates in your diet that you are eating. Your insulin levels get elevated and they stay elevated chronically. Insulin, as it turns out, promotes cancer growth. In fact, when I wrote about this for the *Journal of Science*, I started with the story that this University of Toronto researcher told me why he got involved in this research. He said he had breast cancer cells he was keeping alive in a petri dish in his laboratory.

JORGE: What do they feed the cancer cells to keep them alive?

GARY: You feed them glucose, which is what you get from carbohydrates, and you have to put insulin in the petri dish to keep the cancer cells alive. No insulin, no cancer cells. Breast cells in the human body don't have receptors to respond to insulin, so healthy breast cells arguably don't respond to insulin. But breast cancer cells couldn't live without it. So this researcher got involved in this research. It is pretty clear that insulin is a related hormone to cancer. Insulin is like growth factor hormone—they are tumor promoters. They promote the growth of cancer. Many of the genes that are defective in cancer exist and feed into what is called the insulin-like-growth-factor signaling pathway.

So, the argument is, in effect, that elevated levels of insulin start stimulating the cancer process. And then, basically the cancer cells up-regulate what are called insulin receptors. They get this magnified insulin signal. And insulin feeds blood sugar to them. It helps facilitate the flow of glucose, fuel. Now they start burning more and more fuel. It allows them to multiply and create daughter cells, which is what a tumor does. And it also stimulates their DNA, their genes, and the nucleus of the cell to mutate.

So, this whole process could be driven by elevating insulin levels. And we have good evidence that sugar is responsible. So this fellow, a Harvard researcher (who arguably might win the Nobel Prize someday for discovering an enzyme called PI3 kinase [*Phosphatidylinositol 3-kinases*] that regulates a cell's sensitivity to insulin, and also turns out to be a cancer promoting gene) and another researcher (who is now the president of Memorial Sloan-Kettering Cancer Center in New York, which is one of the three most prestigious cancer research hospitals in the country) both told me that they don't eat sugar anymore.

JORGE: Based on this research?

GARY: In fact, they are actually on something close to an Atkins diet—no sugar, no refined carbs, and a high-fat diet because they don't want to get cancer. Not because they have to control their weight, but because they don't want to get cancer.

JORGE: So if you want to avoid cancer, whether it is breast cancer, prostate cancer, then sugar, hidden sugar, carbohydrates, processed carbohydrates . . .

GARY: . . . are the things to avoid. Not the meat, necessarily. Not the fat, but the refined carbohydrates.

exact same time period. For example, from 1864 to 1900, New York reported a doubling of cancer rates, and in Philadelphia cancer rates jumped from 31 per thousand deaths in 1861 to 70 per thousand in 1904 (more than double). To link it back to diets, consider that sugar consumption in America jumped from 18 pounds per person per year in the 1800s, to an average of 90 pounds per person per year in 1900. In Britain the increase was from 36 pounds per capita in 1850, to over a hundred by 1900. That's how Sugar Calories go to work.

THE PIMA TRAGEDY: THE WESTERNIZATION OF DIETS

Probably the most famous example of what happens when unhealthy Western diets enter pure unadulterated native eating is what happened to the Pima Indians in the 1850s, although similar examples could be given for the Intuits, the Masai, and Samburu nomads, as well as the Australian Aborigines, or Native American tribes. In all cases, when the Westernization of a society happened—the addition of sugar, flour, and white rice—so did obesity, diabetes, and all their not-so-merry mates: cancer, heart disease, and other illnesses. These examples illustrate just how radically sugar calories can and do cause obesity and disease.

The Pima are a Native American tribe in Arizona who, today, have one of the highest rates of obesity and diabetes in the United States. However, until the 1850s, the Pima were known as a hardworking and successful community of hunters and farmers. Reports on the Pima in 1846, described the tribe as in good health, with fine figures, who ate abundant amounts of wild game, fish, and clams—obesity and overweight were not mentioned. In the 1850s, the California gold rush began and tens of thousands of travelers began passing through the Pima territory on the Sante Fe Trail on their way to California. With the gold rush came large numbers of settlers from America and Mexico who hunted the local game to extinction, and diverted the Gila River (which was central to the Pima's fishing and water supply) to irrigate their fields. By the 1870s, the Pima were starving from the invasion and destruction of their land. While they no longer had viable hunting or fishing options, the Pima were still trying to farm what they could, but for the most part, the tribe had become dependent on government rations, which consisted mostly of flour and sugar. In addition, several trading posts had opened on the Pima reservation after the 1850s, and there the Pima purchased sugar and canned goods, which replaced the high protein/low carb components of their traditional diets—and they've never recovered. Along with high rates of obesity, the Pima today have high rates of diabetes and kidney disease.

THE 100 | The Evolution of Diets

Early Insights into Obesity and Overweight

Obesity and overweight became more commonly recognized as a problem in society after the introduction and wide dissemination of flour and sugar. In response, scientists began speculating about causes of such increasing rates of overweight and obesity within more progressive societies as well—and these pioneers were on the right track. In 1844, Jean-Francois Dancel, a French physician and author of *Obesity, or Excessive Corpulence, The Various Causes and the Rational Means of Cure,* wrote: "All food which is not flesh—all food rich in carbon and hydrogen—must have a tendency to produce fat." And, even earlier, in 1825, Jean Anthelme Brillat-Savarin, born in 1755, wrote in the *The*

Physiology of Taste: ". . . a more or less rigid abstinence from everything that is starchy or floury will lead to the lessening of weight." Brillat-Savarin was not a physician, scientist, or chemist, but he was on the right track about diet and obesity. First trained as a lawyer and then a politician, he began writing his opinions about food based on observations of the way in which people ate. He claimed that in the course of over three decades, he had observed dining habits of more than 500 dining companions who were overweight or obese. From these encounters, Brillat-Savarin concluded that "some people, in whom the digestive forces manufacture, all things being equal, a greater supply of fat are, as it were, destined to be obese." To that he added, "the starches and flours which a man uses as the basis of his daily nourishment . . . starch produces this effect [obesity] more quickly and surely when it is used with sugar." This is a pretty amazing observation when you consider the fact that it was made long before gene expressions or even insulin had been discovered.

Still, most doctors in the 1800s until the 1930s touted the conventional wisdom that obesity was a disease and one that was nearly impossible to remedy. Many methods were tried to help people lose weight through these years including eating less, exercising more, leeches to the anus, bleeding from the jugular—all to no avail. "All these plans, however perseveringly carried out, fail to accomplish the object desired [weight loss]," wrote British physician Thomas Tanner in *The Practice of Medicine,* 1869, but he did go on to say, "Farinaceous [starchy] and vegetable foods are fattening, and saccharine matters [sweets] are especially so." While Dancel argued that the doctors who believed obesity to be incurable were prescribing a cure (eating less) that actually caused overeating to occur because it left people in a state of constant hunger. "They forbid the use of meat . . . and direct the patient to eat as little as possible," wrote Dancel, who argued that he could cure obesity if the afflicted person would pass on carbs and eat mostly meat.

These early low-carb advocates were basing their theories on early findings in chemistry (the study of how all matter is composed), and based on these findings, they argued that fat forms in the body from eating carbohydrates and sugars, not protein, and on observations that wild meat-eating animals were never fat, and as Dancel pointed out, if you look to nature, the most obese-looking animals, that is, the hippopotamus, survive on carbohydrates, while the most lean, cheetahs, tigers, and wolves, eat only protein and fat from that protein. The first diet craze was to be born of these wild roots.

Weight Loss Take One

The first diet revolution could be said to have begun in the mid-1800s when one unlikely individual, a wealthy English undertaker, William Banting, found help with a lifelong struggle with obesity. Banting, age 65, weight 202 pounds, in 1862, had been trying to lose weight for nearly 30 years. He had tried a variety of methods: he took up rowing, cut calories, took purgatives and diuretics, consulted the best doctors of the time, tried walking, and horseback riding—all of which failed. Fortunately, Banting didn't give up; he found yet another doctor, the physician, William Harvey, in 1862, and asked for his help. Coincidentally, Harvey had recently returned to England from a Paris symposium where the physiologist Claude Bernard had given a lecture about the harmful role of sugars and starches, and their link to diabetes. Bernard was a pioneer in his own right because he was the first to observe that humans and all living creatures survive by several intricate and interdependent systems in the body that work together for survival (that is, the endocrine system, nervous system, etc.), which we will discuss in detail in the next chapter. What titillated Harvey, though, was Bernard's discussion of how sugars and starches increased glucose in the body—and how this was seen more often in diabetics, who were frequently overweight.

The doctors were guessing (and guessing correctly) that weight gain was linked in some way to the amounts of carbohydrates in the diet because these foods—sugars and starches—were all similarly broken down into glucose in

19TH CENTURY CONVENTIONAL DIET WISDOM: LOW CARB WINS

Near the end of the 19th century, the Congress of Internal Medicine (the premier health agency of its time) met in Berlin to review the most popular dieting methods and trends. Of these, only three were awarded approval as regimens that could be used effectively to reduce weight, the Banting Method and two other diets designed by German physicians. The first program required that even more fat be consumed in the diet than in the Banting food plan, while the second weight-loss plan prescribed leaner meats, fewer beverages, and added exercise recommendations. All three diets prohibited sugar, sweets, and all breads and starches.

The Berlin review on weight loss and the Banting diet initiated numerous variations of the similar diets that would be used for the next several decades across Europe and in the United States.

This same dieting method persisted into the early 1900s. William Osler, a Canadian physician and the founding medical professor at Johns Hopkins, discussed the treatment of obesity in his book *The Principles and Practice of Medicine.* Osler wrote that he advised obese women ". . . to reduce the starches and sugars," and encouraged a diet of mostly protein and fat. Osler also included Banting's eating guidelines, and two other low-carb options by two German physicians, Max Joseph Oertel and Wilhelm Ebstein. Oertel's diet (Oertel was the director of a sanatorium in Munich) restricted fats more than the Banting method, but still featured lean meats and eggs, and included more vegetables and bread. Ebstein, professor of medicine at the University of Gottingen, featured fatty foods because he theorized that they were essential to creating satiety, but he forbid sugars, sweets, and potatoes, and limited bread and green vegetables. Meat, however, was unlimited on Ebstein's plan. All these plans had one thing in common—sugar, which included all carbohydrates, was inherently linked to weight gain.

the body, the same glucose seen in the abnormally elevated blood of diabetics. This is a key point that you'll notice is a common thread throughout this book: *All carbohydrates are in essence a form of sugar.*

Based on this information and Harvey's own theory that diabetes might be linked to obesity because diabetics were almost always overweight, Harvey formulated a diet for Banting that was extremely similar to that of the hunter-gatherer societies described previously, with the exception of beer to drink and a small amount of stewed fruit (which likely hindered even more weight loss for Banting and others who tried the diet). In addition to the ale and fruit, Banting was directed to eat three meals a day of meat, fish, or game, and a small amount of stale toast and tea in the evenings. Within a year, Banting had lost more than 50 pounds, without cutting calories. Banting was so pleased by his success that he wrote a book called *Letter on Corpulence* that was published in 1864, and quickly became a best seller in Britain, Germany, Austria, France, and, a few years later, in the United States. Within a year, the "Banting Diet" became such a craze that it became a verb: to diet, meant "to bant." It is even reported that the emperor of France used the Banting system to lose weight, and did so successfully.

Popular Theories for Treating Obesity: 1900 to 1940

The physicians of the time who implemented the Banting-type diets reported that they were widely successful with hundreds of their patients. The advice—eat meat and fat, avoid starches and sugars—morphed into the conventional wisdom from the 1800s through the mid-1900s and was widely accepted across Europe and in many parts of the United States as well. This was aided by the evolving science that was going on mostly in Germany and Austria throughout the late 1800s up until the Second World War, and these were the people considered the world leaders in the field of obesity research.

Beginning early in the 20th century, the medical research community in Europe, Germany, and Austria began to shift from viewing obesity as simply an incurable disease, to seeing *obesity as a disorder of excess fat accumulation* relating to how fat is regulated in the body. This is critically important because for the first time science was paying attention to the role of genes, long before much science existed for genes or hormones. These physicians were taking note that something was different about fat tissue in the overweight human than in the thin human—just as some people are hairier than others, and some taller than others; some people have a propensity to get fatter than others—something regulated how fat was stored in the bodies of obese humans that was different than it worked in thin ones. Again, this rationale was based on few experimental interventions, and more on observations, and anecdotes reported by those who had success using the method.

This trend can be seen in the recommendations that were published in Europe and in the United States by many physicians treating obesity and overweight during this time, up until the late 1950s (then things began to change, which we'll get into later). In the late 1800s, William Osler, the first appointed physician-in-chief at Johns Hopkins Hospital, revolutionized the medical curriculum in Canada and the United States by synthesizing the research he had learned from his German and British medical education—in essence, he brought the world's theories and knowledge of medical treatment together for the most comprehensive and up-to-date care of the time. His recommendations on obesity were simple, "avoid taking too much food, and particularly to reduce the starches and sugars," as published in his book *The Principles and Practice of Medicine,* in 1901. And, as my mentor, Gary Taubes, points out in his book *Why We Get Fat*, four of the most prominent medical schools, Stanford, Harvard, Children's Memorial Hospital in Chicago, and Cornell, all independently published recommendations for

"Up until this time there had been two competing theories— the calorie imbalance theory vs. the fat imbalance theory. Both ideas shared fairly equal weight among the research community up until the war ended. Today—the idea that obesity is caused by a hormonal imbalance is out, while the idea that it's all about calories in/calories out is *in*."

weight loss from 1943 to 1952, which boiled down to the following seven recommendations:

1. Don't use sugars, including honey, syrup, jams, or candy.

2. Avoid fruits canned with sugar.

3. Avoid cakes, cookies, pies, puddings, and ice cream.

4. Avoid recipes using cornstarch or flour, such as gravies or cream sauces.

5. Avoid potatoes, macaroni, spaghetti, noodles, dried beans or peas.

6. Avoid fried foods.

7. Avoid sodas, including Coca-Cola, ginger ale, or root beer.

And obesity guidelines published in the 1951 textbook *The Practice of Endocrinology* recommended that unlimited amounts of meat, fish, birds, green vegetables, eggs, cheese, unsweetened fresh fruits (except bananas and grapes) be enjoyed; while breads, refined flours, cereals, puddings, potatoes, white or root vegetables, sugars, and all sweets should be avoided completely.

At the same time, another theory on weight loss and diet was born that would eventually shift the low-carb way of thinking out of fashion and into a fad. Louis Harry Newburgh, a professor of medicine at the University of Michigan, published a paper titled "The Nature of Obesity" (1930). In it, Newburgh concluded that the only way to lose weight was to eat fewer calories and to burn more calories. Newburgh's view was that all weight could be controlled simply by restricting calories, or by burning more of them through activity. He also went on to say, rather offensively, that obese people had "perverted appetites" that only needed to be controlled to lose weight. **And that's where the controversy between obesity as a disorder of fat accumulation versus obesity**

as a condition of energy imbalance was instigated, but the controversy was only a newborn at this point. The German and Austrian researchers who believed that obesity was caused by a hormonal imbalance in the body still held weight and were respected. Newburgh's theory was just that—a theory, and both theories existed somewhat equally until a dire turn of events.

When the Second World War began in 1933, the seminal research in Germany and many parts of Europe came to a standstill. The European physicians and researchers who weren't killed, fled the continent, and the pivotal obesity research that had been gaining a firm foothold essentially fell off the map. **Up until this time, there had been two competing theories: the calorie imbalance theory versus the fat imbalance theory. Both ideas shared fairly equal weight among the research community up until the war ended. From that point in time, until today the idea that obesity is caused by a hormonal imbalance is out, while the idea that it's all about calories in/calories out is *in*.**

THE 100 | How Low Carb Fell Out of Fashion

The Fast Track to Fat: 1940s to 1970s

Fast forward to the end of World War II: Thanks to anti-German sentiment in America, the war's abrupt interruption of fundamental German and Austrian research, and the reality that the only funding for obesity research was in the United States, the theory that obesity is caused by a hormonal imbalance dwindled, and was eventually silenced. Decades of research and substantial evidence that carb restricting and avoiding sugar was key to weight loss were simply bypassed for Newburgh's philosophy that obesity is a problem of energy imbalance, and that obese people have a "perverse appetite." **By the 1940s and '50s, Newburgh's theory of eating too much and moving too little emerged as the accepted conventional wisdom that persists today.**

JORGE: I used to be overweight, and I used to always ask myself, what is the problem? What are the actions I'm supposed to take to lose weight? Confirm this for me one more time: What we are told is basically to eat less and exercise more. That is the popular song. Eat less, exercise more.

GARY: We believe it is all about calories. We believe if we take in more energy than we expend we get fat. Therefore, what we are supposed to do is expend more than we take in.

[*We believe this because almost all health agencies, from the American Heart Association, the American Medical Association, the American Council on Sports Medicine, the National Institutes of Health, the Institutes of Medicine, the World Health Organization, and the U. S. Department of Agriculture, to name more than a few, tell us that this is the cause of obesity.*]

JORGE: Makes sense mathematically.

GARY: The math is beautiful, but it doesn't tell you anything about the cause of obesity. That's the problem. Our belief, as the experts have taught us, is that obesity is caused by an energy balance disorder. So it is having more energy in and less energy out. That is the law of thermodynamics. People get fatter therefore you have to pay attention to the energy. This thought dominates all thinking on obesity. It dominates the public health messages: eat less, exercise more. I saw an article in the *New York Times* two days ago. A mathematician from MIH (I mean why anyone would go to a mathematician for help on a physical disorder, I don't know, but they did) said the problem is just too much food available. Remember, we talked about obese populations where the one thing there was that there was not enough food available.

Many of the obese populations I discovered had kids who were starving. You could see it: starving children, obese mothers. But you knew there was not enough food available. So you can find populations where you know that there was not enough food, but there was obesity. How can that be? That goes against everything we believe.

JORGE: Share with us how you would describe the true problem. What were all these people doing back then, in these other countries and today? Why are we fat?

GARY: I can't help but give some historical background. There was always another hypothesis, another way to look at this. It was a German-Austrian hypothesis prior to the Second World War at a time in which the Europeans, the Germans in particular and Austrian clinicians were doing, arguably, the only meaningful medical science in the world. And if you wanted to be a scientist in medicine, nutrition, metabolism, genetics, eccrinology, the study of hormones, or physiology, pre–World War II you had to either speak German, or you certainly had to read it. And if you were really serious, you went to Germany or Austria to work with these people in a post-doctoral position. All the major authorities in the U.S. in metabolism and nutrition had trained with the Germans. So they had different hypotheses. And it wasn't about eating too much or exercising. They said that's silly. You know, it's kind of first principals; obesity is not a sort of energy balance, but of having too much fat. Imagine saying having too much fat is like having too much fat. It is the simplest possible thing you could say. [These scientists knew that something] was responsible for regulating fat tissue. Something must do it. Unfortunately, the Europeans couldn't figure it out by the time the Second World War set in. When the Second World War set in this whole theory—the whole German/Austrian research—vanished with the war. And when the war was over that continent had far more dire problems than trying to figure out what caused obesity.

JORGE: It almost caused it to kind of get buried.

GARY: The whole center of research moved to the U.S. because we had the money to fund research. We got all these young doctors and researchers who, by the way, pretty much hated the Germans.

JORGE: So, anything German, they put it away.

GARY: Yes. This whole literature gets buried and we [the American researchers] create obesity as this whole disorder of energy balance. Actually, eating too much, and psychologists get into the game. And by the 1960s [obesity has become] an eating disorder. Psychologists are studying it instead of physiologists and biochemists, and the people who study fat. The other thing that happened by 1960 is that we had the technology to figure out what does regulate fat tissue. It was the hormone insulin.

Why did Newburgh's theory prevail? This seems to be due to many factors including faulty science following Newburgh that gained biased attention for making fat a dietary evil (this was research done by Ancel Keys, which we'll discuss later in this chapter), politics that favored Keys' faulty science, personality clashes and cliques, food industry involvement and funding of researchers, and journalists whose sensibilities centered on regurgitating without questioning, or at least without reporting both sides of the story—and, as you know, there are almost always two sides to any story. Finally, there seems to be a division to where the relevant research was being put forth—obesity research tends not to cross over into endocrinology and metabolic research, even though they are intimately linked. I'll touch on all these points later in the chapter. For now, let's start with a look at how we became so fat phobic.

INTERVIEW WITH GARY TAUBES

JORGE: From Jenny Craig to Weight Watchers, we have all these solutions that we think work that are, in reality, not working. I have been researching this for 10 years. You have now been doing this work for far more than that. This has been your passion. Tell me what is going on, in your opinion. Is this a modern epidemic? Because it definitely is happening now, and we think it's because of the iPad, and because of computers that we are all sitting too much, and we are eating too much food in general. What are your thoughts?

GARY: The argument today [made by most obesity experts and government health agencies] is that we are getting fat because we don't have enough reason to be physically active, and there is just too much food available. You just can't walk down the street without passing a fast food joint or a convenience store and stopping in, having food, and overeating. So, [we are told] you take in more calories than you expend [and you gain weight].

One of my favorite stories about obesity comes from the 1930s, from a young German physician named Hilde Bruch. Bruch left Germany for America in 1933, when the Nazi party took over. She gets to New York in 1934, and she is stunned. She writes about how stunned she is at the fat kids walking around the streets of New York. And not just fat, she says, roly-poly fat kids. And what is fascinating is this is the heart of the Depression. This is America at its poorest. Something like 40 percent of the workforce or more is out of work. This is bread lines, and soup kitchens, and poverty beyond our imagination. And she is saying that she is seeing these kids who are fat. It was Bruch who started a pediatric obesity clinic at Columbia University, and became the world's leading expert on childhood obesity in the 20th century.

[*Note: Actually, at the height of the Depression in 1933, unemployment was at 25 percent. Although, farmers weren't counted among these unemployed, so Gary's estimates may be closer than they appear.*]

So the argument [that we eat too much, and move too little] for the epidemic, where two thirds of Americans are overweight, and one third are obese, that is new. That dates from somewhere between the late 1970s and early 1990s, but there has always been obesity [in the civilized world]. I point out in my books that you can find populations that have high levels of obesity [among the poor], with rates as high as we have today in the U.S., lots of them, pre-1980s: very poor, no iPads, no computers, no video games, no TV sets, no McDonald's or Burger Kings, and no food industry to speak of.

The point is that if this is what makes us fat, then what was making them fat?

WHAT HAPPENED TO LOW CARB RESEARCH

After World War II, in the 1940s and '50s, the majority of prominent research in Germany and Austria that provided evidence that carb restricting and avoiding sugar was key to weight loss was mostly silenced, with the calories in/calories out argument taking center stage. However, not all such research ceased to exist; it just didn't gain the attention of the public health authorities or the popular media in the same way that Newburgh's theory was gaining traction. Consider the following two studies:

DuPont and the Mostly Meat Diet After noticing that employees were becoming obese, the DuPont Company began diet research in the late 1940s to try to get their employees to lose weight. At first, they tried restricting calories and portions, and to get more exercise, but these strategies failed. So DuPont medicine division director, George Gehrmann, recruited his colleague Alfred Pennington to design a different diet. Pennington prescribed a mostly meat regimen to 20 overweight employees, and they lost an average of two pounds a week, eating an average of 3,000 calories a day. Pennington reported that his subjects reported lack of hunger, increased physical energy, and a sense of well-being. The diet kept carbohydrates to no more than 80 calories per meal.

Pumping up Protein at Michigan State A follow-up to the Pennington diet was done in the 1950s by Michigan State University Nutrition Director, Margaret Ohlson, and her student Charlotte Young. Ohlson and Young put overweight students on calorie-restricted diets and found that they only slightly reduced their weight, and reported feeling lethargic and constantly hungry while on the diet. When the Michigan researchers flipped the diet and had the subjects eat plenty of protein and fat, but only a few hundred carbohydrate calories a day, they averaged a three pound per week weight loss, and they "reported a feeling of well-being and satisfaction. Hunger between meals was not a problem."

Similar findings persisted into the 1970s. Physicians and scientists in Canada, Cuba, France, Germany, Sweden, Switzerland, the United Kingdom, and the United States prescribed variations of carbohydrate-restricted diets to obese men, women, and children. Some plans limited amounts of fats and proteins to certain calorie counts, others prescribed no restrictions at all to meat, poultry, or fish, while they all kept carbohydrates and sugars restricted to some extent. Some diets allowed a set amount of carbohydrate calories, while others allowed virtually no carbs at all, not even greens. In all cases of carb-restricted regimens, the results were similar: Men, women, and children lost weight with little effort and did so without feeling starved.

Heart Disease and Fat Phobia

In the 1950s, scientists took a misguided path that has ultimately led to the obesity epidemic and the diseases of Western civilization that we live and breathe today. In the 1950s, the medical community and the American Heart Association began reporting a tremendous spike in the number of heart disease deaths that were occurring around the world: nearly 50 percent of Americans were dying from heart disease. Also, President Eisenhower had suffered a heart attack in 1955, and for the following six weeks, there were almost constant updates on his health status. These reports mesmerized Americans, but they were misleading in that the increases in reported heart disease had as much to do with new diagnostic inventions (the electrocardiogram in 1918, began to be widely used 1920s to 1950s) and new classifications for heart disease being included on death certificates beginning in 1949, which were happening at this same time. All these factors, media attention about the president, better diagnosis, and more categories, led to the appearance of more heart disease than was the reality. Consider the fact that two new classifications for heart disease were added, one in 1949, and one in 1965—the result was that between 1949 and 1968 the proportion of heart disease deaths attributed to either of these two new categories rose from 22 percent to 90 percent!

Logically, public leaders turned to the heart health leaders of the time—specifically, Ancel Keys, the editor of the American Heart Association's journal, *Circulation*, for answers. Keys, a Harvard and Cambridge educated physicist, had concluded that it was fat in the diet that caused the rise in heart disease based on a study he published based on observations of small numbers of various populations. Keys concluded that people who ate the least fat had the lowest levels of heart disease, and those who ate the most had the highest levels of heart disease. But his findings were flawed.

First, Keys didn't account for the amounts of carbohydrates or sugars any of the populations included in the study were eating as part of their normal diets. Second, Keys only published data using 7 of the 22 countries he actually investigated. In later years when he was called out and his research was reviewed, and all 22 countries were analyzed, no link between heart disease and dietary fat was found—none at all. And, finally, valid research was ignored that opposed Keys. There were studies published during this same time that reliably linked sugar and carbs to heart disease by demonstrating that such foods raise LDL cholesterol and triglycerides. Unfortunately, because the American Heart Association was such an unquestioned leader at the time, these flaws were overlooked. Instead, the message that heart disease was caused by eating fat and fatty foods gained national notoriety in 1956 when representatives from the American Heart Association, including Keys, went on national television to spread their message. With the flawed science widely disseminated, the American public was sold.

This didn't stop researchers and scientists who disagreed with Keys from publishing papers that discounted his findings. And, for the next two decades, many experts provided evidence that the findings were ambiguous and ignored a definitive link between adverse heart health and eating carbohydrates and sugars. Unfortunately, none of the competing evidence made it onto national television or into the popular press, and neither did the data that existed during the 1950s that the prevalence of smoking (known to elevate heart disease) was 50 percent. Instead, the majority of Americans continued to ride the American Heart Association's low-fat wagon that ultimately led us right off the cliff to the obesity epidemic.

The low-fat dogma was compounded in the 1970s when a Senate committee led by George McGovern published "Dietary Goals for the United States," which advised Americans to significantly curb their fat intake, and recommended that more than 50 percent of daily calories should come from carbohydrates. This paper led to the government food pyramid we popularly use today. This is the same food pyramid that has as its base carbohydrates with six to 11 servings a day, and fats as basically a nonentity. The majority of these carbohydrates are made of Sugar Calories, and as you'll learn shortly, these foods cause fat accumulations, and weight gain, even if you try to severely restrict your calories, or exercise for hours a day.

Why McGovern didn't consider the other existing research that was up for

> No human society in history has consumed a diet remotely resembling what the USDA Pyramid suggests as optimal.
>
> —**Nora T. Gedgaudas,** author of *Primal Body Primal Mind.*

debate is unclear, but one factor could have been that he himself was on a low-fat diet at the time of publishing his dietary recommendations, and may have been swayed by his own dietary biases. And then there was the little known reality that the medical community and government agencies in the 1970s and '80s were run by a tight-knit group of Ivy league colleagues, including Keys and McGovern, that had attended the same colleges, conferences, and symposiums, and apparently supported each other, blindly, throughout their careers. Many in this club were also being fed incentives by the sugar industry (see "The Politics of Sweet Matters") that may have helped churn out more damaging findings for fat. There was no questioning what came down from the top, but there was plenty of criticism for anyone who bucked the system. The medical community quickly dismissed diets such as the Atkins Diet Revolution, and research that contradicted Keys was treated as if it didn't exist, or didn't matter.

Over these same two decades, 1950 to '70s, when the theory that eating less and moving more was the only popular solution for obesity, and that fat would kill you, American waistlines continued to expand, and heart disease, cancer, and diabetes increased as well. The flavor of the nation was fat phobic, and fat consumption actually decreased per person over this time period, but our sugar consumption spun out of control.

To meet the demands and marketability of lowering fat in foods while maintaining flavorful options, food manufacturers got busy adding increasing levels of sugars in everything from spaghetti sauce to salad dressings. Labels and packages touted health claims because of low-fat ingredients, while completely forgetting to mention that the fat, that actually wasn't bad, had been replaced by an overload of Sugar Calories that cause weight gain.

"I DID IT!"

CATHERINE

VITAL STATS

AGE: 22 **HEIGHT:** 5' 6" **WEIGHT LOST:** 44 pounds

MY BEST STRATEGY: Trust. I was a complete skeptic when I first started working with Jorge. I was sure that there was no way I could lose weight by having free access to so many foods. I quickly changed my mind when I dropped 12 pounds—in just one week! That turned my attitude around quickly. Here I felt like I'd eaten more food in that first week than I ever had before, but I dropped so much weight. I was a believer, and it hasn't failed me. I also followed the menus to the letter. Jorge makes it so simple because there are no complicated recipes or hard to find foods, but everything is delicious.

The Politics of Sweet Matters

From 1920 to 1980 the rate of sugar consumption per person increased nearly 30 percent and then in the late 1970s high-fructose corn syrup (HFCS) was introduced into the food supply, and by the 1980s our consumption of sweeteners snowballed from 120 pounds a year to over 150 pounds per year per person. We need to take an especially close look at this sweetener, because it dramatically changed the course of our consumption of sugary beverages and foods, and spiked our levels of obesity, but not for the reasons you might think. You've probably heard that HFCS is the supervillain of sugars, but chemically speaking HFCS and most other sweeteners, including table sugars, are not that much different in the damage they do. What makes HFCS especially damaging is that it is cheap to produce and disseminate, its syrupy composition makes

We don't need sugar to live, and we don't need it as a society.

—Dr. Mehmet Oz, a cardiothoracic surgeon, author, and television personality.

it perfect for beverages, and it has a mouth feel like fat (so it can replace fat in foods like french fries).

Remember that fat had been determined to be criminal to our health from the 1960s onward, and the unfortunate result was a free pass to sugar. The food industry started pumping out many low-fat foods that were laden with sugars because sugars are fat free. In addition, the sugar industry and makers of HFCS quickly began funding research that was looking into the role of dietary fat and obesity. These weren't exactly unbiased participants.

The warping of the health advice we've received over the years is as disturbing as it is perverse. Beginning in the late 1950s, after dietary fat had been vilified, and avoiding anything padded with it was the popular dogma of the day, the Corn Products Company, the makers of Mazola margarine, initiated programs to "educate" doctors that the polyunsaturated fats in corn oil would lower cholesterol and prevent heart attacks. The company also collaborated directly with the American Heart Association on releasing a handbook for physicians to raise a butter-is-bad awareness. Now I know that this is a fat for fat throw down, but corn oil is another cheap commodity that the food industry loves to push, and margarine contains truly terrible hydrogenated fats that are akin to eating plastic and do hurt your heart health, while butter actually won't hurt you at all. In the next chapter, I'll explain all of this in detail. By the 1970s, the influential public health officials who touted the low-fat dogma were accepting money from private donations from the likes of General Foods Corporation (maker of Post cereals, Kool-Aid, and Tang), Oscar Mayer, Coca-Cola, and the National Soft Drinks Association. By pairing politics, personalities, and manufacturers of sugar and carbs a severe threat was leveled against finding a real solution for obesity and overweight—all because the solutions being touted miss the real point: that carbs and sugar (Sugar Calories) drive the hormone insulin, and insulin drives overeating and the storage of fat in our bodies.

INTERVIEW WITH GARY TAUBES

GARY: The sugar industry loves this idea that it is all about calories. They argue it all the time.

JORGE: Is it true that sugar is the only food that isn't regulated by the government? I mean folic acid, vitamin C, fats, and proteins, there is an allowance of sorts. But is there one for sugar?

GARY: Well, the sugar industry has always worked actively and behind the scenes to make sure that [the government] never puts a cap, a max amount, on sugar consumption.

Despite the fact that over the last 50 years, sugar consumption has tripled in the U.S., the government's Dietary Guidelines for Americans still advises only that sugar should be used in moderation.

Now, the sugar industry comes along, and there is science in the 1960s implicating sugar as well. There was a famous British nutritionist named John Yudkin who said sugar is the problem. It is not fat. It is sugar that causes heart disease. It is sugar that causes diabetes. You can show it in animals. You can show it in young subjects.

JORGE: You can prove it.

GARY: Not only prove it, but we can demonstrate [sugar's role]. The sugar industry had to respond to this. People had taken seriously the idea that sugar causes diabetes. Type II diabetes wouldn't exist if we didn't eat sugar. Doctors are taking it seriously. So the sugar industry did hire scientific consultants who said you have to study [sugar's role in disease and obesity]; it's important. [The consultants recommended spending] as much money as possible on large clinical trials to figure out if [sugar was] killing people. But instead of doing that [the sugar industry decided] to do some public relations. So they put together a food nutrition advisory committee with some of the money. And they start this committee with scientists who believe that dietary fat and cholesterol are the problem.

JORGE: So fat and cholesterol are the bad guys?

GARY: You have two competing ideas. One says it is sugar. One says it is fat and cholesterol. Because you are selling sugar, you get your advisory committee stocked with people who believe the problem is fat and cholesterol. You put out a report saying the problem is fat and cholesterol, not sugar and then you disseminate the report. One of them disseminated like 25,000 copies of this publication called "Sugar in the Diet of Man" written by all of these major scientists.

JORGE: Which sounds very credible.

GARY: The biggest for sugar was the founder and chairman of the Harvard Nutrition Department, a guy named Fred Stare, who was exposed in 1977, but by then all the damage was done.

[*Fredrick John Stare was one of the best-known nutritionists in the United States. He founded the Department of Nutrition at the Harvard School of Public Health in 1942 and served as chairman until he retired in 1976. He was the founding editor of the journal* Nutrition Reviews, *wrote a nationally syndicated column for many years entitled "Food and Your Health," and published several popular books on nutrition.*]

JORGE: Exposed for?

GARY: Exposed for taking huge sums of money from the sugar industry and from other processed food manufacturers. Stare just thought it was part of his job. I don't think he was venal. He just thought, "My job is to take money from industry and protect industry." That is what he thought nutrition people were supposed to do. And he was probably venal, too.

[*The nutrition center Stare was in charge of took money from General Foods Corporation, the maker of the very carbohydrate-rich Post cereals, Kool-Aid, and Tang breakfast drink. His department also took funds from the sugar industry and companies like Oscar Mayer, Coca-Cola, and the National Soft Drinks Association.*]

Stare was a very good-looking, charming guy. Very lean, so he probably thought, although he is actually quoted in an article saying he doesn't eat sugar because he prefers to save those calories for his nightly martini. So this combination, [the sugar industry got] people who believed fat was the problem to advise them, they wrote the reports for [the industry] exonerating sugar. Then those reports, when the FDA got around to deciding whether sugar should be considered safe, they got all these journal articles, apparently annotated, referenced documents saying there is a little bit of evidence implicating sugar, but there is a lot more evidence exonerating it—all written by these guys who thought fat was the problem. Then the FDA says, you know, it is all kind of ambiguous. We are going to decide that sugar is fine.

To make matters worse, HFCS was seen as a healthier alternative because it didn't spike insulin the way that table sugar did. (In the next chapter, we're going to dissect the science underlying why both of these sweeteners, and almost all caloric sweeteners, are similarly fattening.) Plus, HFCS was less expensive to produce, so it was used rapidly and widely in virtually all sodas and many other foods. In a USDA report published in 2005, authors write that "Americans have become conspicuous consumers of sugar and sweet-tasting foods and beverages. Per capita consumption of caloric sweeteners (dry-weight basis)—mainly sucrose (table sugar made from cane and beets) and corn sweeteners (notably high-fructose corn syrup, or HFCS)—increased 43 pounds, or 39 percent, between 1950–59 and 2000. In 2000, each American consumed an average 152 pounds of caloric sweeteners; 3 pounds below 1999s record average 155 pounds. That amounted to more than two-fifths of a pound—or

The inescapable fact is that certain people are making an awful lot of money today selling foods that are unhealthy. They want you to keep eating the foods they sell, even though doing so makes you fat, depletes your vitality, and shortens and degrades your life. They want you docile, compliant, and ignorant. They do not want you informed, active, and passionately alive, and they are quite willing to spend billions of dollars annually to accomplish their goals.

—T. Colin Campbell, a nutritional biochemist and researcher, and co-author of *The China Study*.

JORGE: So, why are we fat, Gary?

GARY: So, we think of insulin as a hormone that is missing in dysfunctional diabetes. Insulin keeps blood sugar down and controls your blood sugar. Also, one of the ways it controls your blood sugar is by sticking fat calories and carbohydrate calories in your fat tissue, and keeping them there. So by the 1960s you should have had this hypothesis that obesity is a disorder of insulin signaling, just like diabetes. And, in fact, some of the obese people are diabetic, and so many diabetics are obese that you would think of them as two versions of the same disease. There are researchers who refer to them as diabesity. And they are both disorders of insulin signaling. **And here is the key—we secrete insulin primarily in response to the carbohydrate content of the diet. The more carbs, the less fat in the diet, the more insulin you secrete.** The more sugar in the diet, the more we become what is called insulin resistant. This is what the research from the 1960s showed, this is what is being recapitulated now. So, you could argue that it is refined carbohydrates, which are the ones that you digest easily; so refined grains, starches, and sugars will cause obesity in susceptible people.

JORGE: And not just white sugar, could be sugar from any source?

GARY: High-fructose corn syrup and fruit juices. Any form that you find sugar in a form that is easy to digest. So here is the kicker: It is that basically flour and sugar are the cause of obesity. Now you can explain what was going on with those poor kids in New York in the 1930s. Well, they were poor and they were not getting a lot to eat, they were living on starches and bread.

JORGE: That is what they were fed in New York City in 1930?

GARY: The bread kitchens—I mean literally bread lines. You were literally living on potatoes, bread, and sugar. Back then, ice cream was new, soda was new, candy was new. That is what was driving obesity. When you are poor, you can't afford to eat a lot of meat. Green vegetables are virtually nonexistent in these poor communities. So what you get are easily digestible starches and sugars.

America's sweet tooth increased 39 percent between 1950–59 and 2000 as use of corn sweeteners octupled

Item	Annual averages					
	1950–59	1960–69	1970–79	1980–89	1990–99	2000
	Pounds per capita, dry weight					
Total caloric sweeteners	109.6	114.4	123.7	126.5	145.9	152.4
Cane and beet sugar	96.7	98.0	96.0	68.4	64.7	65.6
Corn sweeteners	11.0	14.9	26.3	56.8	79.9	85.3
High-fructose corn syrup	.0	.0	5.5	37.3	56.8	63.8
Glucose	7.4	10.9	16.6	16.0	19.3	18.1
Dextrose	3.5	4.1	4.3	3.5	3.8	3.4
Other caloric sweeteners	2.0	1.5	1.4	1.3	1.3	1.5

Note: Totals may not add up due to rounding.

Edible syrups (sugarcane, sorgo, maple, and refiner's), edible molasses, and honey.

Source: USDA's Economic Research Service.

52 teaspoonfuls—of added sugars per person per day in 2000." The obesity epidemic follows this same trajectory.

The Obesity Epidemic: 1980s to 2012

By the 1980s and '90s, the government would declare an obesity epidemic was upon us.

Remember that this spike in weight coincided with the lowering of fat in the diets, while raising the consumption of sugars and carbohydrates in the daily food patterns for most people. We've been taught to think of carbohydrates as different from sugars, but it's important to realize that all forms of carbohydrates are simply and ultimately sugars. Regardless of the food (potato or ice cream) your body turns the carbohydrate into a sugar (glucose) so it can be processed. Some carbs are better than others of course, and I'll explain all the details of this in the following chapters, but it's important to realize that all carbs are really sugars—which is why I call them Sugar Calories—but our government agencies have always separated the forms of sugar into carbohydrates and sugars. Certain sugars are healthier based upon several other factors including

- processing

- refining

- vitamins, minerals, antioxidants

- water content

- fiber

Basically, after the actual sugar is taken into account, the amount of processing and refinement that a food goes through (what it takes to get from an apple to apple juice, or from a beet to table sugar, or a grain of wheat to wonder bread), the amount of nutrients that remain in the food, the water content (a carrot or watermelon versus a raisin or a hard candy), and, most importantly, the fiber a food has. Fiber is especially important because your body cannot digest it, and it helps shuttle out bad calories as well. More on this later—for now it's back to the history lesson.

"The public health authorities told us unwittingly, but with the best of intentions, to eat precisely those foods that would make us fat, and we did. We ate more fat-free carbohydrates, which, in turn, made us hungrier and then heavier. We are in the midst of an obesity epidemic that started around the early 1980s, and that this was coincident with the rise of the low-fat dogma. (Type 2 diabetes, the most common form of the disease, also rose significantly through this period.) They say that low-fat weight-loss diets have proved in

JORGE: Everything we are doing in today's world is based on science that is logical and mathematical. It should make sense. It is mathematical science on weight loss. It is about eating less and exercising more, but we know that based on the results that this logic doesn't work. The majority of our culture, of our world, the Western world is overweight. It is an epidemic that is going to overburden health care.

GARY: There is a line from Robert Lustig, the pediatric obesity expert in San Francisco.

[*Robert Lustig is a pediatric endocrinologist at UCSF and a professor of clinical pediatrics. Lustig came into the public arena because of his arguments about fructose's adverse effects on humans. On May 26, 2009, he delivered a lecture called, "Sugar: The Bitter Truth," which was posted on YouTube the following July and went viral with some 2.5 million viewings; see it at http://youtube/dBnniua6-oM.*]

He says that before you can have any serious healthcare reform you have to have obesity reform. Obesity, diabetes, and Alzheimer's; the three of them are going to take down the healthcare system. You have to figure out what is causing them. We can't blame it on the fat people. We can't just say they aren't listening to us. They aren't paying attention. We have to accept the possibility that we are doing the wrong thing—and we are doing the wrong thing because we have the wrong perception of what causes the disease. If this were still the AIDS epidemic instead of the obesity epidemic, if young men, homosexual men were still dying by the hundreds of thousands per year you would question if you understood the nature of the disease correctly. But obesity experts don't. They [public health officials, obesity experts, nutritionists] insist that it has to be about calories. However, if you turn it into a biological issue instead of a physics issue, instead of a mathematics equation . . . and ask, what regulates our fat tissue? What stimulates those hormones that put fat in our fat tissue? Now you are implicating specific products in the American food supply.

clinical trials and real life to be dismal failures, and that on top of it all, the percentage of fat in the American diet has been decreasing for two decades," writes Gary Taubes, author of *Good Calories, Bad Calories.*

While the percentage of obese Americans stayed relatively constant through the 1960s and '70s at 13 percent to 14 percent, it then spiked by 8 percentage points in the 1980s, and by the 1990s nearly one in four Americans would be obese. Meanwhile, overweight children nearly tripled in number, and physicians began diagnosing what used to be called adult-onset diabetes in adolescents (it had to be renamed Type 2 diabetes because of how prevalent it has become in children). Interestingly, the rise in sugar consumption coincides with rising obesity rates, 20 percent from 1970 to the 21st century.

THE 100 | Conclusion

Today, 68 percent of Americans are obese or overweight. The predominant message from health officials, the medical establishment, and obesity researchers is that fat is bad, low fat is good, and the only way to lose weight is to cut calories, and to move more. We are also taught to believe that we should consume more than half our daily calories from carbohydrates (let alone the other hidden Sugar Calories in their other recommendations), but as I already mentioned above, while we're encouraged to get some of those from whole grains, we're never told that all carbohydrates are actually sugars—some better, some worse—and controlling Sugar Calories is the key to losing weight.

I know this is a lot of information to digest, but now that we've reviewed the historical concepts that have brought us to our current state of affairs, it should be clear that the excess pounds you struggle with are a result of your trying to follow the recommendations as dictated. The conventional wisdom for losing weight that exists today has set you up to fail, but not for lack of

Time period	Key events
2 million years ago to 10,000 years ago	10,000 years ago humans began farming, which introduced starchy vegetables such as potatoes, corn, rice, and beans.
10,000 years ago to 1700s	Agriculture and refining flours and sweeteners were perfected. Overweight and obesity first noted by archeologists and anthropologists.
1700s	Sugar and flours available to the wealthy. These foods were considered "clean," and "healthy" because they didn't spoil like fresh, natural foods.
1800s	Health experts identified starchy and sweet foods as the cause of weight gain. Low-carb diets were conventional wisdom. First published papers on obesity, dieting, and cures.

Banting diet introduced. Mass refinement of sugars and flours completed mid-1800s, making both widely available. |
1900–1940s	Competing obesity theories: obesity is a disorder of fat accumulation vs. obesity is a disorder of energy imbalance.
1950–1970	Heart disease in the news; fat is a dietary evil, sugar consumption spikes, carbs become the basis of a healthy diet, obesity increases.
1970–1980s	Introduction of HFCS, identification of obesity epidemic, carb and sugar consumption continues to increase.
1990–2012	Obesity continues to be epidemic, sugar consumption has leveled off, but carbs continue to be pushed as the foundation for the food pyramid and a healthy diet. No one knows that carbohydrates are actually sugars in disguise.

willpower or sincerity on your part. You can try to follow these recommendations until you are blue in the face; they won't work because they inherently go against how your body is genetically designed to handle food. The key to getting on the right track, as I mentioned at the beginning of this chapter, is to trace our steps back to find ways of eating that match our genetic blueprint. This is fantastic news because that's just how I've crafted The 100, and in the

INTRODUCTION OF MODERN FOODS

THE BIG BAD BOYS

Distilled alcoholic beverages 800–1300

Refined sugar (widely available) 1850s

Refined grains (widely available) 1850s

High-fructose corn syrup 1970s

Food	Date	Food	Date
Saltine crackers	1876	Oreo cookies	1913
Best All Purpose Pillsbury Flour	1881	Moon Pie	1917
Coca-Cola	1886	Milky Way	1923
Log Cabin Syrup	1888	Wheaties	1924
Fig Newtons	1891	Kool-Aid	1927
Triscuits	1895	Rice Krispies	1928
Tootsie Rolls	1896	Hostess Twinkies	1930
Graham crackers	1898	Fritos Corn Chips	1932
Wesson Oil	1899	Kraft Macaroni & Cheese	1937
Chiclets Chewing Gum	1900	Kit Kat bar	1937
Hershey's Milk Chocolate Bar	1900	M&M's candy	1941
Karo Corn Syrup	1902	Cheerios cereal	1945
Pepsi-Cola	1902	Frozen orange juice	1946
Campbell's Pork & Beans	1904	Instant mashed potatoes	1946
Peanut butter	1904	Cheetos	1948
Kellogg's Corn Flakes	1906	Frosted Flakes	1952
Hershey's Kisses	1907	M&M's Peanut Candy	1954
Quaker Puffed Wheat	1909	Fruit Loops	1963
Mazola Corn Oil	1911	Doritos	1966
Hamburger buns	1912	Pringles Potato Crisps	1969

Source: Adapted from www.geocities.com/foodedge/timeline.htm.

"I DID IT!"

LESLIE

VITAL STATS

AGE: 41   **HEIGHT:** 5' 4"   **WEIGHT LOST:** 17 pounds

MY BEST STRATEGY: Be persistent. Tenacity, resolve, determination—these are the characteristics that have helped me get through the tough spots. Sticking to my goals through thick and thin has given me results that have been worth the effort. In the office where I work, there are almost daily temptations, from donuts, pastries, and bagels, to cookies, chocolates, and candies. And if not those treats, it is almost always someone's birthday, wedding, or baby shower. I never used to even think about it, I just grabbed a fork and a napkin and dug in, until I met Jorge. With his way of eating, I have learned to free myself from sugar, and to prepare so that I don't fall in the treat trap anymore. This program has changed my life, and it's changed my daughter's life, too, because I've been able to show her how to eat in a healthy way. This program can be done without struggle, and it can fit any lifestyle.

following pages you'll learn that it's a way of eating and living in the modern world that is molded to match your biologic needs. The result is that you drop pounds effortlessly, all the while feeling happy, content, and energized.

I hope that your eyes are now open, so you can shift your perception to what really makes a body healthy and slim. Just for a moment, consider that almost everything you've been told about weight loss has been completely backward. You don't have to believe it all yet, but do allow yourself to think about the ideas I've presented here. With the knowledge you've obtained in this chapter you now know that a calorie is not a calorie, but that some calories count and some don't. You've been misled, misfed and kept in the dark regarding the true history behind the obesity epidemic—we all have—but no more! Now the light of knowledge illuminates your path so you can take control of your health and well-being. With this newfound sound wisdom laying a solid foundation, you are on your way to shedding pounds with my revolutionary method that, once and for always, puts sugars where they belong. Get ready to live the path that will keep you slim without feeling starved.

Contemplate the life-changing value of the information you've just read and get ready to go deeper. In the next chapter, I'll take you further into the Science of Skinny so that you'll fully understand the mechanics of your body, the role that Sugar Calories play, and how some foods cause fat storage and accumulation, while others burn it off effortlessly.

The Science of Skinny

To say "you are what you eat" is wrong.
You are what your body does with what
you eat.

—ERIC WESTMAN, DUKE UNIVERSITY

W hy does anyone become obese? Conventional wisdom would have you believe that it's all about numbers—you become obese by eating too many calories, and burning off too few, but as we began to explore in the previous chapter, it isn't that simple. In this chapter you'll gain a deeper understanding of how it isn't the calories you ingest versus the calories you expend that determines weight, but a much more complex system orchestrated by the body's chemical messengers and determined by the quality of food choices you make (not by the quantity of food you eat). By the end of this chapter you'll not only understand the true cause of obesity, but also what we do as a society that continues to exacerbate the obesity epidemic, and what steps need to be taken to turn things around for good. When you understand the mechanics that cause your body to store excess fat, and how sugar is the main culprit in obesity and disease, you'll fully comprehend the mechanics that cause your body to burn excess fat and the ability to lose weight and keep it off long term.

In the last chapter, we laid the historical foundation—how humans progressed from lean hunter-gatherers to the modern-day plagued-by-obesity society we are today. By following the changing dietary habits, and the political and public health messages we've been fed you've begun to get an idea of how certain foods cause weight gain, and how certain recommendations exacerbate it. Now, we'll again look at changing dietary habits, but this time we'll do it from a different angle—the scientific one. In the last chapter, you learned how the introduction of refined carbohydrates and sugars coincided with the rapidly increasing rate of obesity. On the following pages we'll get more into the workings of your body to learn, from the inside out, what happens to the foods you consume—how our bodies ingest, burn, and store different elements that make up different foods—and how this is relevant to obesity, overweight, and disease. By the end of this chapter, you'll clearly see how our struggle with excess poundage isn't caused by the number of calories in your daily diet, or by the lack of calories displayed on your treadmill each day, but by the Sugar Calories you eat.

> **"What really determines the number on the scale, and changing it, is the type of food you choose to eat and how your body reacts to that food."**

First, I'll discuss the mechanics involved in running a balanced healthy body, from a biological context, so you can clearly see the factors that contribute to how the human body is made to regulate weight including how fat cells work in the body. You'll see how the body is much more than a gas tank that can be simply filled with fuel and then run until empty. It's a complex system that communicates with the foods we eat to determine how they should be stored and regulated. Most important, you'll learn all about the hormone that determines where all fuel goes in the body, and how it controls your fat cells. Understanding how insulin works, and how it regulates fat storage is the key to unlocking weight loss that lasts long term.

Next, we'll take a look at what causes a body to be thrown off balance—not only what causes weight gain and obesity—but also what makes you vulnerable to conditions and diseases such as diabetes, heart disease, cancer, and Alzheimer's.

> "You'll see how the body is much more than a gas tank that can be simply filled with fuel and then run until empty. It's a complex system that communicates with the foods we eat to determine how they should be stored and regulated."

Sugar is the common and insidious thread you'll see throughout these conditions. Once you understand the science behind what causes disease and obesity, what nutrients a body really requires, and what makes a body glom onto excess weight you'll be able to see how backwards it is to try to lose weight by cutting overall calorie intake, reducing fat, or exercising more.

Finally, I'll discuss why most diets and exercise fail to produce long-term results, how your brain reacts to sugars and refined carbs to create the cravings that sabotage your best efforts, and the way you can eat for the rest of your life to be healthy. In other words, how to get your body back to a balanced state.

It can be a real "Aha!" moment when you see how we've all been attacking this obesity thing in a backward manner, and that's exactly what I want you to experience. I want this information to empower you to take charge of your health and well-being, and to prime you for the following chapters where you'll learn the key to Sugar Calories, and the secret to handling all foods, so you are set you up for success.

The Human Body in Harmony

The balanced body is a beautiful thing. If you want to hold the key to unlocking "thin," first you must be able to see how all the parts of the body are meant to work in unison, almost exactly the way the New York Philharmonic Orchestra together is a beautiful harmonic ensemble.

— "I DID IT!" —

ABBY

VITAL STATS

AGE: 40   **HEIGHT:** 5' 6"   **WEIGHT LOST:** 54 pounds

MY BEST STRATEGY: This way of eating isn't a gimmick or a fad. You don't overthink on this program, so it isn't overwhelming. There are no special products or vitamins you have to purchase. I treat my cravings like the addictions they are—I take every meal one at a time. I say to myself, "I don't have to eat this way forever. I am eating this way for the rest of the day." **I also found it essential to give up artificial sweeteners. It's the only true way to lose the taste for sugar, and the cravings that go with it.** In reality, my fear of giving up diet sodas was much worse than actually doing it.

Just as a symphony needs its conductor to direct and guide all the sections to work together—the woodwind, brass, percussion, and strings sections—to make beautiful balanced music, your body's weight-regulating system has a top down hierarchy that tells it what to do. If one section of the orchestra is too sharp or flat, it can throw the whole sound off; if the conductor isn't in tune with the orchestra, he might misdirect a section and throw off the whole beat—it can be a fiasco without the right finesse. Similarly, your body needs a healthy conductor with a well-tuned and trained orchestra to create its own beautiful music.

Our conductor, the hypothalamus, lives in the base of our brain and works by sending out and receiving chemical and nerve messages that tell the body what to do and how to react. The hypothalamus works with several interdependent systems including the endocrine, nervous, digestive, circulatory, respiratory, immune, reproductive, skeletal, muscular, and integumentary (the skin, hair, and nails) systems. When all systems are go, our bodies work in a beautifully balanced state—for example, our circulatory and respiratory systems maintain a set temperature (98.6°F) by setting off internal cooling (sweating) and heating (shivering) functions; our immune systems (our disease-fighting centers) have plenty of white cells ready to keep enemies at bay; and our digestive system and circulatory system helps us process the food we eat into the appropriate amount of fuel we need. It's this last system we want to take a closer look at to understand how the mechanics of getting fat work.

> "If you want to hold the key to unlocking 'thin,' first you must be able to see how all the parts of the body are meant to work in unison almost exactly the way the New York Philharmonic Orchestra together is a beautiful harmonic ensemble."

The body's chemical messengers are its hormones, enzymes, and nerve impulses that work together to send signals back and forth across the systems mentioned above to regulate all systems of the body, but the one that trumps them all is the hormone insulin. Insulin is to the hypothalamus what the first violinist is to the conductor. The leading first violinist is the concertmaster of the orchestra. Your hypothalamus communicates directly with your endocrine system, which is the system that controls all the chemical messengers that tell your body what to do (via hormones).

The endocrine system has four functions: 1) controls reproduction, 2) regulates growth and development of all cells, 3) maintains the internal environment (temperature, hydration), and 4) regulates energy production, utilization and storage. This last function, which controls the first three, is controlled by insulin, which is secreted from the pancreas. This is important for us to note because it links insulin with the regulation of energy (insulin tells your body what to do with the food you eat), how to use this energy, and how to store it.

The Master Hormone

Historically, insulin's role relating to fat storage and weight gain wasn't understood. Initially insulin was thought to be responsible for only removing and storing sugar in the blood.

The first step to better understanding how insulin worked in the body began in the early 1900s by experts who were studying diabetics. While the condition of diabetes had been known for hundreds of years by its symptoms—excessive urination, unquenchable thirst, weight loss (type one diabetics), and death—insulin's link to diabetes was discovered in 1921 by Frederick Grant Banting (no relation to William Banting from the last chapter), an orthopedic surgeon, and Charles Herbert Best, a medical student. Banting and Best were able to first replicate diabetes by removing the pancreas from dogs, which caused a dramatic spike in blood sugar and other diabetic symptoms. The researchers then cured the condition by figuring out how to isolate and inject insulin that they created from dried portions of dog pancreas back into the canine that had previously had its pancreas removed. Once they figured out that insulin was produced by the pancreas it wasn't long before the two scientists were able to cure a boy with diabetes by injecting insulin that had been extracted and isolated from a dog pancreas as well, and soon after that insulin was being marketed and used in hundreds of diabetics. By 1978, a way of making synthetic insulin from human origins was discovered, and has been used with great success ever since.

> "Insulin is the main regulator of fat storage and mobilization, and how all energy in the body is disseminated."

What does this have to do with gaining weight and fat accumulation? While insulin was first recognized for its effect on blood sugar and diabetics in the mid-1920s, the other significant outcome noticed with insulin therapy was weight gain. "The fact that insulin increases the formation of fat has been obvious ever since the first emaciated dog or diabetic patient demonstrated a fine pad of adipose tissue, made as a result of treatment with the hormone," wrote Reginald Haist and Charles Best, in *The Physiological Basis of Medical Practice*. In fact, *insulin therapy* was so good at producing weight gain that it became a popular treatment for anorexics during the 1920s and '30s. The doctors who used the therapy in underweight individuals noted that insulin caused patients to have voracious appetites and to crave and eat large amounts of carbohydrates.

This realization eventually led to the understanding that insulin is the main regulator of fat storage and mobilization, as well as how all energy in the body is disseminated. In many ways, insulin determines how fat or thin you will be. By the late 1960s, scientists knew that injecting insulin caused dramatic spikes in hunger, increased carbohydrate and sugar consumption, and rapid weight gain. There were also tests available at this time that would show that the more obese a person, the higher their insulin levels.

Today we know that insulin . . .

- Regulates fat, carbohydrates, and protein metabolism.

- Enhances the storage of fats in fat cells.

- Inhibits the release of fatty acids from storage.

- Signals proteins and molecules to repair and grow cells.

- Signals fat cells to pump in blood sugar (glucose), which is turned into glycerol, and then is bundled into heart harming triglycerides. Triglycerides are the stubborn fat that is hard to move back out of your body.

- Creates new fat cells if the ones we have are getting full.

- Signals liver cells to make fatty acids into triglycerides where they can be stored in fat tissue.

- Triggers metabolism that converts carbohydrates into fatty acids in the liver and inside fat tissue.

For an in-depth illustration of how insulin works on a typical lunch see "Lunching on Insulin." Unfortunately, the role of hormones was only vaguely understood in the early 20th century, and linking hormones to obesity was rejected outright by Newburgh—the leading obesity expert of the time–which perpetuated the idea that weight gain was simply a numbers game, while ignoring the fact that when certain hormones (specifically insulin) are triggered by certain foods (carbohydrates) fat storage is increased.

INSULIN'S HELPERS

Insulin is responsible for how our bodies store fat, but it doesn't work in isolation. Two primary enzymes that are influenced by insulin dramatically affect how fat is stored and how fat is burned in your body: lipoprotein lipase and hormone-sensitive lipase.

Lipoprotein lipase (LPL) is an enzyme that lives on the exterior of liver, fat, and muscle cells. One function of LPL is to grab fat from the bloodstream and shunt it into fat cells. When insulin is running high in your body (in response to eating carbs), it signals the LPLs on fat cells to grab up as much fat as possible from your bloodstream and to store it away in fat cells. These same LPL enzymes on muscle cells are suppressed by insulin, which signals your body to burn blood sugar and store away fat. If you only eat fat and protein, it won't spike your insulin, so it won't cause LPL to do the fat-shuffle.

Hormone-sensitive lipase (HSL) is an enzyme that helps liberate fat from fat cells, and ideally makes you leaner. This molecule lives inside fat cells. HSL's job is to break down triglycerides (bulky fats inside fat tissue and the liver) so they can be used as fuel. Insulin, in even small amounts, turns off HSL enzymes, which in turn causes fat cells to hold on to fat instead of burning it as fuel. So, if you eat a high carb meal, it spikes your insulin and tells your cells to hang onto fat.

To illustrate what happens to the food you eat, and how insulin controls what happens, let's look at a typical lunch: Imagine you are standing in line at your local deli to pick up an Italian ham and cheddar sub sandwich with lettuce, tomato, and mayonnaise—just thinking about the sub is making your stomach growl. Already your body is behaving just like those dogs in that old experiment with Pavlov and his bell—your thought of your sandwich is your bell, and in response your brain sends a message that causes your digestive juices to be stimulated, and alerts your pancreas to release the hormone insulin so it will be ready to regulate the food that is coming in. Next, you get your sandwich, pay the cashier, and take your first delicious bite. Your meal contains refined simple carbohydrates in the Italian roll; fats in the mayo, cheese, and ham; protein in the ham and cheese; and complex carbohydrates in the lettuce and tomato. As you begin your first bites your pancreas pumps out more insulin in response to the rise in blood sugar from the food you are eating. Because carbohydrates are the fastest burning fuel, the insulin tells the fat and protein to get out of the way (these nutrients get shuttled off to your cells)—like the conductor of the orchestra who might tell the percussion section to wait until it is needed—the insulin in your body tells the fat and the protein to wait in storage in fat, liver, and muscle cells while the carbs in the meal are burned off first. If you'd made this meal a salad instead of a sandwich, your insulin wouldn't be spiked, and your cells wouldn't be told to store fat.

But alas, the insulin tells your muscle and liver cells to store this fuel as glycogen (a form of glucose), and some may be converted to fat (especially if there are too many carbs in your meal), and your fat cells store the glucose as fat. As you continue to eat, your blood sugar drops and so does your insulin—then and only then can fat from your cells be released. The lower your carb intake the faster your body can get to using fat for fuel.

Here's how author Gary Taubes outlines the 11 step chain of events in his book, *Why We Get Fat*, which happens in your body from first bite to last.

1. You think about eating a meal containing carbohydrates.

2. You begin secreting insulin.

3. The insulin signals the fat cells to shut down the release of fatty acids (by inhibiting HSL) and take up more fatty acids (via LPL) from the circulation.

4. You start to get hungry, or hungrier.

5. You begin eating.

6. You secrete more insulin.

7. The carbohydrates are digested and enter the circulation as glucose, causing blood sugar levels to rise.

8. You secrete still more insulin.

9. Fat from the diet is stored as triglycerides in the fat cells; some of the carbohydrates in your meal are converted into fat in the liver.

10. The fat cells get fatter, and so do you.

11. The fat stays in the fat cells until the insulin level drops. If you consistently eat too many carbs (Sugar Calories), this never happens.

As you can see, insulin works to increase the fat you store and decrease the fat you have available to burn. Insulin makes us fat.

The Fat Factor

So now you understand how insulin increases fat in the body. But what about fat itself? What is fat and why does it exist?

Fat tissue, or cells, exist in our body to protect our organs and to keep us warm. It used to be thought that fat tissue was also for long-term storage, so that if we were ever starving we would have fuel in reserve to burn off, but now we know this is incorrect. Fat cells have a distinct structure and are interlaced with blood vessels that closely connect to capillaries, which means fat cells can take up fuel and burn it (blood vessels and capillaries are how fuel gets into and out of cells). In fact, fat cells can be responsible for 50 to 70 percent of our fuel needs in a typical day. There is a 24-hour cycle to fat—you start accumulating fat at the beginning of your day, and then, ideally, you burn off the fat between meals, and when you go to sleep at night. That's why you start out at your lowest weight in the morning and gain weight all day. The food choices you make throughout your day will affect how well this system works. The more carbs you eat, the more insulin is increased; the more insulin is increased, the less fat is used as fuel.

It helps if we think of the food we eat processes through our body like the way kids, and sometimes dads, play with Lego. When you get a new Lego set there is several packages of Legos and instructions on how to build up the Lego set. As you open each set and follow the instructions you begin to have your new figure take form. If you do it right you end up with a beautiful figurine. Do it wrong and you end up with pieces stuck in the carpet, under the couch, and sometimes in the next room; to me, that is life's mystery. Let's apply this to how your body works. The proteins and fats in your meal are similar to the packages. The missing pieces is how insulin affects your meal. As you sit down to enjoy your healthy and nutritious meal full of proteins and fats you are essentially building your body back up, restoring all the parts to be a beautiful new you. If you then add these insulin stimulating foods you are essentially losing some of the building blocks into your fat storage areas, carpet, couch or in the next room. This process of missing Legos is how we start storing fat. There are two types of fat in the body, fatty acids and triglycerides. To take the above analogy a step further, we can compare these two fats to the missing Legos. The fatty acids are like the Legos in the carpet and under the couch because they are still fairly accessible to a point. The other fat, triglycerides, are like the

Legos way over in the other room. These bulky fats are made of three fatty acids linked together by a glycerol molecule; they are meant to be for long-term storage. Triglycerides are too big to be freely used as fuel, and it is these fats that are the most stubborn and dangerous to our bodies. Think about it: Your body cannot use the entire lego set if there are missing pieces. Insulin is like your young child scattering Legos all over the house, and generally it isn't until we have used all the building blocks that we start to look for these missing pieces.

INTERVIEW WITH GARY TAUBES

GARY: Back in the 1960s, we buried this idea that insulin regulates fat accumulation. Today when someone is told that they are fat because they eat too much or they exercise too little; there isn't any discussion about what regulates the fat tissue. I could be 300 pounds and as a doctor you are telling me it is because I eat too much. It is like you aren't concerned about the biological factors that are regulating this huge accumulation of fat. If that was a tumor, and there are people who have 200 pound cysts, in that case all you care about are what hormones are causing it. You might take it out surgically, but what hormones and enzymes and broken genes are involved in the growth of this tumor? But when it is fat tissue, you don't care. As long as people think of [weight gain] as calories you don't think about it in terms of regulation.

JORGE: So what is the shift in thinking we need to get to better understand obesity?

GARY: Well, again, [that obesity] is a disorder of too much fat accumulation. You can just say, okay, what is regulating this? If you were walking down the street or sitting in a café, and a guy walks by who is 8 feet tall, the first thing you are going to say in your head is "Whoa, too much growth hormone." It doesn't matter if he is 300 pounds. He probably will be if he is 8 feet tall.

JORGE: So we immediately think his height is due to hormones, not because of overeating.

GARY: Due to hormones. But the same guy walks by who is 6 feet tall but weighs 400 pounds and we think, "What a slob. No will power. Doesn't exercise enough." It never crosses your mind to think, "Boy, too much insulin."

JORGE: So, Gary, if it is too much insulin, does that come from too much sugar?

GARY: It is because of this idea it is all about calories. We've been taught that it is all about gluttony and sloth. Eating too much, exercising too little—this kind of biblical idea merged with this mathematics, physics idea. The other reason is in the 1960s we started to believe that dietary fat causes heart disease. So, if fat causes heart disease, you tell people to eat low-fat diets and you replace the fat with carbohydrates. So then you are telling people to eat high-carb diets. And, in fact, the same carbohydrates that, for instance, my mother's generation believed were fattening—pasta, bread, rice, potatoes—were transformed into heart-healthy diet foods in the 1960s. That is why the base of the food pyramid—pasta, bread, rice, potatoes—is what it is, because [these foods] don't have fat in them so you can eat them as much as you want [according to the low-fat philosophy]. They will protect you from heart disease.

SPECIAL SUGAR: ALCOHOL

Alcohol is another special carbohydrate that is mostly processed by your liver. For example, 80 percent of the calories in a shot of vodka go straight to your liver where it is converted into a small amount of energy and into a molecule called citrate. Citrate fuels the conversion of glucose into fatty acids—the end result is an increased production of fat in your liver (see the FAQs on page 217, for more information).

HOW INSULIN INCREASES FAT

To get a clearer understanding of insulin's role in making, accumulating, and storing fat inside our fat cells let's consider the following three facts:

1. Inside every fat cell are enzymes that are made to burn fat (called hormone-sensitive lipase or HSL)

2. On the surface of every fat cell are enzymes that shuttle in fat from the bloodstream (called lipoprotein lipase, or LPL)

3. Fat cells are covered with capillaries that can shuttle in blood sugar to be turned into fat

So what does this have to do with insulin?

When insulin is triggered from a meal including too many Sugar Calories it:

1. Shuts off fat burning enzymes

2. Turns on fat storing enzymes

3. Signals blood sugar to be shuttled into the fat cell to be turned into fat

When you eat a meal that is rich in protein, fat, and vegetables your insulin remains low, which as a result:

1. Keeps your fat burning enzyme burning fat

2. Shuts off your fat storing enzyme

3. Prevents blood sugar from elevating

4. No signal is given by insulin to shuttle it into your fat cells

MISUNDERSTOOD: CHOLESTEROL

Cholesterol—the fat in our body—has several components. The way we've been taught to understand the various mechanisms of our cholesterol and its effects has been misinterpreted by our public health leaders, and misrepresented by drug companies. Most of us have been taught to think that fat is bad because of guidelines that tell us that fat in the food we eat raises our cholesterol, which in turn raises our risk of heart disease, and will make us fat—but it isn't true.

You've probably heard of cholesterol in the following ways: First there's your good cholesterol, or high density lipoproteins (HDLs); then there's your bad cholesterol, or low-density lipoproteins (LDLs); and finally, there's the worst cholesterol, the triglycerides. Usually included in this overly simplified description is the explanation that eating fat in your diet increases the bad fat and lowers the good fat, while eating carbohydrates is good for lowering the bad parts of cholesterol. This is not only incorrect; it is just plain backward in almost every sense.

LDLs (bad cholesterol) aren't actually bad, as we've been told; it depends on the density of the LDL. If it is small and dense it is a problem, especially if it has been damaged by oxidization. Free radicals damage the LDL and make it stick to the inside of the arteries making them very dangerous. The large and fluffy LDLs are not. That's right, there are two different types of LDLs. Small is bad, large is good. Bad LDL is created by elevated insulin and overconsumption of refined carbohydrates and sugars. Good LDL is created by the fat in your diet. Without carbs to spike insulin, the fat you eat actually makes much fluffier LDLs that appear to be harmless. Eating healthy omega-3 fat also increases your HDLs—the good cholesterol—and lowers your triglyceride risk, while sugar and highly refined carbs (again with the Sugar Calories) decrease HDLs and increase triglyceride formation in your body (see "Sucrose and Fructose: The Most Fattening Carbohydrates" on page 61 for more information).

While Americans have dutifully reduced the percentage of daily calories from saturated fat since 1970, the obesity rate during that time has more than doubled, diabetes has tripled, and heart disease is still the country's biggest killer.

—Melinda Wenner Moyer

The Elevated Insulin Epidemic

Putting together what we've discussed so far—how the body is meant to work in a state of balance, how insulin and carbohydrates can throw off this balance, and how fat cells can become influenced to be more for storage than for fuel—prepares us for this section: How elevated insulin, caused by out of control, and misunderstood, sugar consumption, is responsible for the obesity epidemic.

Our society, thanks to an excessive overload of refined sweeteners and carbohydrates, has generated a culture of people who have consistently elevated insulin levels. This is what is driving our fat epidemic and what, in the end, drives all imbalances when it comes to disease and illness.

Here's how it works: When insulin remains abnormally elevated over time (from eating toxic levels of sugar), your cells decide they don't want it (they become resistant). When this happens, the blood sugar sticks around in the bloodstream; this triggers the pancreas to pump out more insulin, which tells your fat cells to suck up the excess blood sugar. When this pattern is repeated over time, your body turns into an elite fat-storage system, and becomes resistant to letting go of fat, making it nearly impossible to lose weight. Another interesting tidbit about insulin resistance is that not all cells become equally resistant at the same time, or in the same way, and this can cause us to store away excess pounds as well. Part of this occurs as we age. Your muscle cells are the first to go, getting more and more resistant to insulin, while your fat tissue stays more sensitive for a longer period—that means that your fat cells will still be good at storing fat, but your muscles won't be as good at burning fuel or staying strong.

Insulin resistance also increases the production of triglycerides (the body's stubborn bulky fat), and lowers HDL cholesterol (the good cholesterol), which in turn increases blood pressure, zaps your energy, and makes you feel fatigued.

Having elevated insulin can also happen in the womb. This isn't just a problem that is isolated to the individual who eats too much sugar and carbohydrates—we are actually evolving to create more fat people by continuing to eat diets that keep insulin elevated. During pregnancy, the pancreas feeds the developing fetus—and if a mother's diet is high in carbohydrates, it will drive insulin in the pancreas, which will drive insulin into the fetus. Therefore, women who have high insulin levels are at risk for giving birth to babies with an already insulin-enhanced system, making the next generation even more vulnerable to carb cravings, and fat storage. That's why some of us may be programmed to store fat—we were manufactured for it in the womb.

Overweight and Obesity

When all this information is taken into consideration, it's easy to see how obesity is a disorder of fat accumulation caused by the overstimulation of insulin, which is caused by our modern-day high carbohydrate and high sugar diets. This way of eating sets up a vicious cycle of hunger, overeating, and over-storing of fat. The overall calories in our diets don't cause our weight gain; the types of foods that drive our hormones to store fat instead of burning it do. This is why calorie-restricted diets and exercise ultimately fail. Increased levels of insulin will make you fat and make sure that you *stay* fat. To paraphrase George Cahill, a former professor of medicine at Harvard and an insulin expert, "Carbohydrate [sugar] is driving insulin is driving fat."

Our modern-day diets cause our insulin levels to remain abnormally spiked preceding diabetes by one to two decades and by the time someone becomes a diabetic it may be too late to reverse the damage (this is one of the reasons that obesity is linked to type 2 diabetes), and anything that causes insulin to remain abnormally elevated will increase the period throughout our days when fat is being told to stay stored, and decrease the period where we can burn fat.

This imbalance causes obesity, and it causes all the other conditions commonly known as the diseases of Western civilization.

Sucrose and Fructose: The Most Fattening Carbohydrates

To understand where our equilibrium was knocked out of whack, we need to look at some sweet matters: carbohydrates. Ultimately carbohydrates, which I more accurately refer to as Sugar Calories (this includes all grains, starchy vegetables, flours, and caloric sweeteners), determine insulin secretion, which drives the accumulation of fat, and therefore obesity. All carbohydrates—yes, even whole grain breads, potatoes, and apples—are made into glucose (your body's sugar) in your body, and therefore increase blood sugar, which causes the same chain reaction that sugar does. And while there's good argument for limiting all carbohydrates, it is also true that not all carbohydrates are created equally.

The most fattening of all carbohydrates are the most highly refined and processed sweeteners: table sugar, high-fructose corn syrup (HFCS), and the liquid and refined carbohydrates we get in the form of sodas, fruit juices, and other sweetened beverages (the majority of these are sweetened with HFCS, which I'll discuss a little later). Next in line are the refined grains sweetened with aforementioned sugars: cookies, cakes, crackers, chips, breads, pasta, and cereals. These products are virtually devoid of fiber, minerals, and vitamins. And, finally, the starchy grains including potatoes, corn, and rice. And lastly fruits. In this section, we'll focus on the first two because they are the most

Not only does eating too much sugar lead to obesity, diabetes, and tooth decay, it is also one of the biggest contributors to low energy and feelings of being overwhelmed—it has even been scientifically linked to depression.

—**Dr. Frank Lipman,** founder and director of the Eleven Eleven Wellness Center in New York City.

harmful and ubiquitous sweeteners in our diets. All the above foods contain high amounts of Sugar Calories. Without a firm grasp on how Sugar Calories work, and how they need to be limited, you'll struggle to lose weight and keep it off. Almost all other carbohydrates can be worked into your diet safely by following The 100™, which I'll discuss in chapter 4.

The problem with table sugar and HFCS is that we eat too much of both, and their chemical compositions are toxic to our bodies in several ways. Luc Tappy, PhD, a fructose, diabetes, and metabolism expert and biochemist from the University of Lausanne, Switzerland, describes the issue this way: "With the exception of a limited amount of free glucose and fructose present in honey and fruits, grains and other starchy food have been the sole source of carbohydrate in the western diet for the major portion of man's history. Sucrose [table sugar] is not only a nonessential dietary element, it has two undesirable consequences. First, because of its rapid digestion, it leads to surges in blood glucose that may place some stress on the homeostatic mechanisms [the body's system of balance] mediated by insulin; and second, it introduces fructose, which we do not need and whose metabolism, when ingested in excessive amounts, imposes an important metabolic burden on the liver."

Let's break it down. Table sugar is made up of 50 percent glucose and 50 percent fructose, while HFCS is 55 percent of the former and 45 percent of the latter. These sweeteners deliver a double whammy to our bodies. To get an idea of how these ultra-fat enhancing carbohydrates work let's look at what happens when we drink one of America's favorite beverages:

You drink a soda sweetened with HFCS (remember it is 55 percent fructose and 45 percent glucose). The glucose goes directly into your bloodstream, spikes your blood sugar, and signals your insulin. The fructose, on the other

Sugar is a type of bodily fuel, yes, but your body runs about as well on it as a car would.

—V. L. Allineare, writer.

hand, can't be transformed into glucose, so it goes to your liver where there are enzymes to metabolize it into fat—triglycerides, specifically. Once transformed, the fat is shipped over to your fat tissue for storage. Since fructose doesn't become glucose in the bloodstream—it's transformed into fat first, and then transported by low-density lipoproteins (LDLs), which are fats, so they don't spike blood sugar, or signal insulin. But remember the glucose portion of HFCS—thanks to that insulin is spiked, turning your fat cells on to storage mode, so most of that soda and anything you ate with it is put in your fat cells, and made into those stubborn triglycerides that don't like to budge. Table sugar works in almost the same way.

Because the average American typically consumes 22 teaspoons of added sugar or HFCS per day, that's around 88 grams (the average teenager trumps that by having 36 teaspoons or 144 grams per day), the majority of us have insulin levels that are abnormally elevated much of the time. This also doesn't include the Sugar Calories that the average individual gets from the other carbohydrates in the diet, just the added sugar calories. Over time, this excessive intake of sugars in our diets—whether it's from donuts, granola bars (often sweetened with HFCS), chips, sodas, fruit juice, spoons full of sugar in our coffee, or sports drinks—and the longer these foods are part of our eating regimen—the more our bodies keep insulin elevated, the more resistant our cells become to the insulin, which makes our poor pancreases pump out ever more insulin, which causes more of the energy we eat to be converted to fat. Plus, our livers are overworked because they are creating more and more triglycerides from the fructose we are consuming and shipping off to our fat cells, where fewer and fewer of these triglycerides are broken down and allowed to escape from our fat cells to be used as fuel to burn. The result is that 68 percent of humans are overweight or obese, and plagued with diseases such as diabetes, heart disease, cancer, and more.

One other truly sad thing about fructose is that many people back in the 1970s and '80s, when HFCS was first introduced, got the message that fructose was a healthier sweetener, because it was touted as the sugar found in fruit, "fruit sugar," which it is, but the concentration in fruit is in much lower concentrations, and mixed with nutrients, fiber, and water. For example, in a cup of blueberries there is only a small percentage of fructose. When, in its early stages, fructose was mistakenly thought to be so healthy that it was promoted to those with diabetes because it didn't spike blood sugar—that advice reversed when the adverse load to the liver was discovered. Surprisingly, even today you can still purchase fructose sugar (when I searched on Google Shopping recently I got more than 10,000 hits!) and it is touted as a healthy food to boot. One search result even boasts a "65% lower blood sugar response than regular sugar," and says it is "for use in a low-glycemic diet." Anyone who doesn't know the science behind how fructose is metabolized into fat might be fooled into eating this very unhealthy fattening sweetener. In fact, did you know that the touted healthy, all natural, sometimes organic, sweetener agave nectar is basically another form of concentrated fructose?

The Other Sugar Calories:
Refined Carbohydrates and High Sugar Starches

White flour, white rice, white bread, white pasta, corn flakes, chips, Cheese Doodles, crackers, instant oatmeal, and so on—all these foods have one thing in common—they have been highly processed and refined, and are read by your body as sugar. In nature, most grains and legumes naturally contain fiber, vitamins, and minerals—and even those on the low side here, tend to be bulkier (unmilled oatmeal for example)—all of these things lower the elevation effect of insulin. The refined carbohydrates have been stripped of all the "healthy" from nature, just like sugar, leaving you with an empty powder or product that raises your blood sugar, and drops it, almost as quickly as refined sugars do. That's why I've included these foods, as well as the highest starch/sugar foods including potatoes and many fruits on the Sugar Calorie list. Because these are foods that act to spike your blood sugar, and in response, your insulin levels, they must be tracked just as refined sweeteners are—eaten freely, these Carbohydrate Sugar Calories will sabotage your weight loss goals.

In the end, it's the overconsumption of all Sugar Calories in the diet that are highly linked to obesity, overweight, diabetes, cancers, heart disease, Alzheimer's, and many other chronic diseases common to the civilized world (see "Diseases of Western Civilization" on page 66).

THE 100 | How Conventional Wisdom Fails

Why Exercise and Diets Fail

First, let's look at exercise: One reason that exercise doesn't work as a weight-loss strategy is that it makes us hungrier, so whatever fuel you burn off during a workout you gain right back by eating more afterward. Also, remember LPLs (the enzymes that tell your cells when to store fat)? Well, during exercise, as you increase your energy expenditure, LPL enzymes are increased on muscle cells—telling them to hold on to their fuel—and LPL drops on fat cells telling them to burn the fat. It looks good at first, but after your workout, LPL reverses what it is doing—muscle cells shut off their LPL, while the LPL in fat cells shoot up to restock the energy you've just used up. This is one of the reasons that you feel hungrier after your spin class. It loops back to insulin because insulin regulates LPL: The higher the insulin in your system (after a workout), the more LPL on your fat cells are activated so more fat is pulled in and stored—while the same insulin suppresses LPL on muscle cells and tells your body to burn sugar. I'll discuss exercise more in chapter 9 on page 193.

Now for diets: We've already discussed one of the reasons why diets that rely on cutting overall calories and fat fail—insulin's response to carbohydrates and sugars. But there's another side that is often discussed by experts as the

DISEASES OF WESTERN CIVILIZATION

As we discussed in the last chapter and earlier in this one, there was a time when humans were pretty much disease free. Scientists have found that the cause of virtually all chronic diseases, such as cancer, diabetes, heart disease, and Alzheimer's—to name a few—was caused by the dietary shift that happened over the last two million years, with the most dramatic change happening 200 years ago with the introduction of refined foods high in sugar and carbohydrates.

Metabolic Syndrome In the 1980s, a Stanford diabetes expert Gerald Reaven described a collection of symptoms that were common to obesity, diabetes, and heart disease and named them Syndrome X (this was later renamed metabolic syndrome). The symptoms include high levels of triglycerides, low levels of HDL cholesterol (the good cholesterol), high blood pressure (hypertension), chronically elevated insulin (hyperinsulinemia), insulin resistance, and glucose intolerance (an inability to metabolize blood sugar properly). As you'll see below, the effects of insulin and carbohydrate consumption affect the increase of diabetes, heart disease, and obesity—and therefore increase the chance of metabolic syndrome.

It's hard to ignore the fact that highly refined, easily digestible starches and sugars are the culprit in almost every incidence of disease—and that metabolic syndrome seems to be the granddaddy of diseases. Our diets are chronically and consistently high in sugars and refined flours, which dramatically increases our body's blood-sugar load, insulin spikes in response and becomes chronically elevated, and our tissues become resistant. And the high concentrations of fructose in HFCS and other sugars cause our livers to be flooded, and your liver in turn overproduces triglycerides. Our bodies are out of balance because of these very recent changes to our diets.

Type 2 Diabetes Insulin resistance, discussed earlier in this chapter, is the main precursor to type 2 diabetes. Once you have it, you're well on your way to getting type 2 diabetes, according to Harvard researchers who linked the chronic consumption of sugars to an increased risk of diabetes. Other scientific studies published by the American Heart Association and the American Diabetes Association have described how excess fat, especially belly fat, dumps fatty acids and hormones into the liver, which causes it to make excessive amounts of glucose—which, again, elevates your insulin levels and in turn causes insulin resistance, leading back to type 2 diabetes. This broken cycle causes your pancreas to work overtime producing ever more insulin and wearing it out—when your pancreas can't work as it should, and your cells have been flooded with chronically elevated amounts of insulin they fail to respond, and you have type 2 diabetes. This condition makes you more vulnerable to all sorts of other health conditions including vision loss, heart disease, depression, nerve damage, gum disease, skin problems, circulation issues, and stroke. Type 2 diabetes can reduce life expectancy by almost 15 years, and causes more than 70,000 annual deaths.

Cancer Excess sugar consumption causes an increased risk of pancreatic cancer, according to Swedish researchers who found that individuals who consumed more sugar-laden foods and sodas were more likely to get this deadly cancer. Sugar consumption and increased colon cancer risk was reported on in a study published by the *Journal of the National Cancer Institute*, and researchers in Italy identified a direct association between breast cancer rates and eating sweet foods. Cancer cells love glucose, which is what your body breaks food down into so that it can be used as the fastest burning fuel. The more you eat highly refined sugars and carbohydrates, the more you fuel cancer cells. This is all frightening stuff. An overproduction of insulin, caused by excessive consumption of sugars has also been linked to an increased risk of breast cancer. Cancer takes more than 550,000 lives per year.

Heart Disease Overweight women who consumed meals that were high on the glycemic index (high in easily digestible, highly refined, carbohydrates and sugars) were 79 percent more likely to develop heart disease than overweight women who ate the least amount of these highly refined foods, according to a study published in the *Journal of the American College of Cardiology*. Dutch researchers speculate that these trends may be explained by the effects that a high glycemic-index diet has on blood glucose, which can stimulate fat production and inflammation, reduce insulin sensitivity. Inflammation causes your arteries to swell and stiffen, which causes problems in circulation. Diets high in Sugar Calories also raise the amounts of small dense LDLs that can block the flow of blood in your arteries. To make matters worse, as discussed previously in this chapter, triglycerides are a main cause of heart disease, and eating a high sugar diet increases the levels of the heart harmful fats. Drinking just two sodas a day (79 grams of sugar) can increase your heart disease risk by 35 percent, according to researchers from the Harvard School of Public Health. Cardiovascular disease takes more than 600,000 lives every year.

Fatty Liver Disease When you eat lots of foods containing fructose, table sugar, or high-fructose corn syrup, your liver is overrun with the sweetener—fructose can't be managed by your bloodstream as discussed above—and it can cause your liver to literally turn to fat. The liver can only process so much fructose and other sugars into triglycerides and then transport them to the fat cells—if you have too many in your system you begin to have a build up of fat droplets in your liver. This is what happens to force-fed geese in the making of foie gras—in us it is a predisposing factor to getting type 2 diabetes.

Aging High blood sugar can also attach to proteins in the bloodstream and create modified proteins called advanced glycation end products (AGEs). In a study published in the *Journal of Nutrition*, researchers found that excess consumption of Sugar Calories is linked directly to increased amounts of AGEs. The more AGEs you have in your body, the faster the actual aging processes can occur. That means wrinkles people. The most susceptible AGEs are collagen and elastin, which are essential in keeping your skin smooth and supple. Sugar will literally streak and sag your face with lines and loose skin.

Immune Health Your disease-fighting system can't do its job when your diet is overloaded with Sugar Calories. This is because the white blood cells that are the soldiers of your immune system are impaired by refined carbohydrates and sugars. Experts at Loma Linda University in Southern California found that sugars impaired neutrophils (the main type of white blood cells you have in your body) from conquering bad bacteria for up to 6 hours—the main job of the neutrophil along with gobbling up viruses.

psychology of obesity. That's the part of the diet where you can't overcome cravings or stay motivated, so you fall off the wagon and binge. This has often been blamed on willpower, but there is a biological basis for cravings as well—and once again it is related to insulin.

In calorie-restriction diet studies, several patterns emerge that explain why the diets fail. Consider the results of the following studies:

- **You'll feel constant hunger and cold, and you'll regain the weight.** In 1944, University of Minnesota researchers put 32 men on a six-month calorie-restriction diet. The men ate just under 1,600 calories a day of mainly bread, potatoes, and cereals with token amounts of meats and dairy products. Prior to the study, the men had been eating about twice as many calories. In addition to the diet, the men were required to walk an average of five miles a day. At the three-month mark, the men had lost an average of 12 pounds, and by the end of the study, they had lost, on average, 15 pounds of fat. Along with weight, the men reported a host of adverse effects including constant hunger, feelings of weakness, loss of ambition, depression, irritability, and a pattern of feeling cold. When the study ended and the men were able to return to unrestricted eating they found that their appetites were insatiable and their food intake rose as high as 8,000 calories a day. They all regained weight and body fat, eventually weighing on average five percent more than they had before the study started—and they gained 50 percent more body fat.

- **You'll lower your metabolism (the amount of calories your body burns at rest).** In a more recent study, published in the *New England Journal of Medicine* in 1995, researchers from Rockefeller University found that calorie restriction resulted in reduced energy expenditure, constant hunger, and a lower metabolism (the subjects burned lower amounts of the calories they were eating). These subjects also regained the weight lost during the trial.

- **You won't lose weight.** In a 2002 review by the Cochrane Collaboration that looked at the results of calorie-restriction diets (also called appropriately, semi-starvation diets) and low-fat diets, the researchers concluded that neither strategy was successful. They concluded that the weight loss achieved on either type of diet "was so small as to be clinically insignificant."

- **You won't maintain any weight you do lose.** In another review in 2001, when researchers from the U.S. Department of Agriculture analyzed 28 low-fat diets (20 were also calorie-restricted diets), they found that the subjects didn't maintain any weight loss successfully—and in one case the subjects actually gained an average of a pound.

In a chapter on obesity in the *Joslin's Diabetes Mellitus,* written by Harvard Medical School investigators, it states that calorie-reduction diets are "difficult to accomplish despite a wide variety of specific dietary approaches." People, and you know this if you've been on any diet that cuts calories, can't withstand how they feel on these diets for any length of time, and ultimately they lead back to overeating and gaining back even more weight. While many experts today realize that these types of diets don't work, surprisingly it is still the number one method for losing weight that is recommended.

Why Calorie Counting Doesn't Work

Have you ever wondered what the heck a calorie actually is? We sort of take them for granted—the USDA bases all our recommended daily nutrients on a 2,000-calorie diet, while various weight-loss programs will prescribe you a certain calorie count per day depending on your height and weight, 1,600 to 1,800, and other severe food-restrictive programs even put the obese on a paltry 800 calorie per day diet. As of 2011, as part of the Obama Health Care Initiative, all large restaurant chains in the nation are now required to put calorie

JORGE: What should the federal government do about the obesity epidemic?

GARY: We have to act. The public health authorities know we have to act. There is no doubt about that. We have to stop it.

JORGE: What could happen or what is most likely to happen if this trend with the obesity epidemic continues?

GARY: Right now, the estimate is around 150 billion dollars is spent yearly in the healthcare system on obesity and its associated chronic diseases, and that number will double by 2030. It is a huge amount of money going to obesity care, and treating these diseases. It is overwhelming the health-care system. You can make the argument as I have that as obesity and diabetes increase they also increase cancer rates. They probably increase Alzheimer's and dementia rates, too. So if you can lower these numbers you can take an enormous strain off the healthcare system.

JORGE: How do we lower the numbers?

GARY: That's the catch, what do you do about it? Things are getting worse and worse. We have been giving the same advice for 40 years; eat less, exercise more. There are a lot of inconsistencies they [*the proponents of conventional wisdom*] never think about because then they have to confront their assumptions. You get more zealous with your message. [*It's like talking louder to someone who speaks another language—it just doesn't work if you aren't speaking the correct dialect.*]

JORGE: That is where we are at right now.

GARY: That is where we are at right now.

[*Here, Gary is talking about how the experts who came up with the theory that the solution to obesity is in energy expenditure, are resistant to questioning the effectiveness of this theory. No one likes to admit that they may have been wrong, and Gary is saying that the experts are not immune to this.*]

The alternative is [admitting that] maybe "we" got the message wrong, or "we" understand this wrong. And if we do that, we have to accept the possibility that we have been giving the wrong advice for 40 years. Cognitive dissonance is the psychological term. People don't like cognitive dissonance. They very well know that the way to deal with cognitive dissonance is to ignore all evidence that suggests that your beliefs are simply wrong.

JORGE: It reminds me of when we thought the world was flat. I mean is that the last crazy, big idea.

GARY: There have been a lot of crazy, big ideas. There are certain people who think nutritionists can't be wrong. They think the scientific community—all these smart people can't get it wrong. We have this history over and over and over again of very smart people getting it wrong. I mean smart people get it wrong all the time. Ideally, they get it wrong a little less often than less smart people because they put more thought into that.

information on their menus and drive-through signs. So now you know that your Grande Vanilla Latte and your Morning Bun from Starbucks will empty your pocket of $6.30, while filling you up with 600 calories. The same legislation requires that vending machines post calorie content as well, so you can no

With the lack of light in winter, we are naturally drawn to comfort foods that elevate our mood and raise our blood sugar. There are very real, physiological reasons for this. Remember those famous scenes in the *Golden Girls* when Blanche, Sophia, Rose, and Dorothy got up at night and ate cheesecake to feel better? Sugar elevates the neurotransmitter beta-endorphin, a brain chemical that is akin to opium and morphine. Sugar consumption actually dulls pain and makes us feel better, but only temporarily! Then it leads to systemic inflammation, the root cause of heart disease, diabetes, and some cancers. It can also cause your skin to look horrible and any aches and pain to feel even worse.

—**Dr. Christiane Northrup,** board-certified OB/GYN, who specializes in women's health, and has authored several books including *The Wisdom of Menopause* and *Women's Bodies, Women's Wisdom.*

longer hide from the 275 calories in a Twix. On the one hand, having access to these calories can be helpful, and will certainly aid you in the later parts of this book when you begin tracking your Sugar Calories, but they leave out an important piece of information—not all calories count!

Ah, but I digress from the initial question posed at the top of this section. So then, what is a calorie? A calorie is simply a unit of measurement for heat; in science, a calorie is defined as the unit of heat required to raise 1 gram of water 1 degree Celsius. The term found its way into the food world around 1890, when the USDA used it in a report on nutrition. Back in the day, when scientists needed to figure out the calorie counts in foods they would actually set them on fire, then put them in water, and then check the change in temperature to determine the calories in a certain food. These scientists used a device called a bomb calorimeter, which calculates the change in heat from an ignited food in a closed container. In high school chemistry lab experiments, this is sometimes done with a covered coffee can (that has been separated into two compartments with foil) and a thermometer. By burning food in one compartment, and having water in the other, you can measure the temperature change of the water before and after the fire, and determine the calories from that. What you are really measuring is the amount of energy lost to the fire (this energy would be "lost" to your body if you ate the food). Since the food is lit up in a closed container the heat can't escape, and it raises the temperature in the water.

Today, scientists and chemists use a more precise measuring process to determine calories that take into account the specific amounts of moisture, fats, carbohydrates, and proteins of foods, but the description above paints the general picture. From all this measuring, scientists today know that the following is true for the major macronutrients:

> "Back in the day, when scientists needed to figure out the calorie counts in foods they would actually set them on fire."

- one gram of fat contains 9 calories or heats 9 degrees Celsius

- one gram of protein equals 4 calories or heats 4 degrees Celsius

- one gram of sugar contains 4 calories or heats 4 degrees Celsius (carbohydrates are actually forms of sugar)

Therefore, the amount of calories in any food item is equal to the amount of (fat * 9) + the amount of (protein * 4) + the amount of (carbohydrate * 4) (in grams). For example, in a chocolate kiss, which contains 1.3 grams of fat, 0 grams of protein, and 3.6 carbohydrates the equation would go as follows:

(1.3 g fat)(9cal/g) + (3.6 g)(4cal/g) + (0 g)(4 cal/g) = 26 calories. Ta da!

So now you know what a calorie is—and all our problems with obesity would be easily solvable if our bodies worked just like an incinerator—throw in the food and whoosh, we'll just burn up that fuel. The problem is that each one of us is unique and our bodies do various things with different components in foods, and have different reactions based on these different foods, meaning that two foods with identical calorie counts can have radically different effects on your body depending on the composition of the food.

For a clear example, let's take a quick look at one normal-size Reese's Peanut Butter Cup, which has 105 calories, and let's compare it to the same number of calories in a handful of dry roasted peanuts (about 18 peanuts equals 105 calories). They should be exactly the same right? Not so quick. When you take a closer look at the composition of these two foods you can see that the candy has 12 grams of carbs, with 10.5 of these being sugar, which equals 48 calories of carbohydrates (remember a carbohydrate gram is worth 4 calories). These are the calories that spike insulin and cause fat accumulation and resistance to releasing fat from the body. (These are the Sugar Calories, in the next chapter I'll explain how to calculate for them.) The peanuts, on the other hand, have just 3.9 grams of carbs (a mere 0.8 of a gram of sugar), which equals just 15.6 insulin-stimulating calories—not enough to cause fat storage to be triggered. The peanut butter cup has more than three times the amount of weight-causing calories than the peanuts.

That's why, when it comes to the calories in highly refined, easily digestible carbohydrates and sugars (the Sugar Calories), these are the foods that must be counted. In contrast, the calories in fats and proteins don't spike blood sugar or insulin, which is why these calories don't count in the same way. In fact, they help your body burn fat as fuel, and let go of stored fat. These are your Freebies—the proteins and fats that keep insulin levels low, as do leafy greens (and some other vegetables) because of their fiber and low amount of natural sugars.

I'm not saying that you can eat 5,000 calories of meat a day and stay slim, unless perhaps you are Michael Phelps, but within reason—and a lot of leeway—you can eat comfortably by following The 100™ guidelines (coming up in the next chapters) and still lose weight, and keep those pounds off long term.

INTERVIEW WITH GARY TAUBES

JORGE: The truth is based on what has been given to the world from the media, scientists, and from the government. It truly isn't the fault of the overweight or obese person, is it? The government, the media have been misleading.

GARY: We've been getting the wrong advice our whole lives. It is worse than that. Obese people try arguably harder than lean people to eat the right foods, do the right things, and follow advice. They struggle their whole lives.

"I DID IT!"

ALLISON

VITAL STATS

AGE: 43   **HEIGHT:** 5' 7"   **WEIGHT LOST:** 28 pounds

MY BEST STRATEGY: Don't think of shedding pounds as only getting into your skinny jeans. Weight loss is about so much more than just looking better, and when I remember that it's about health, energy, and confidence I'm way more motivated than when I just watch the scale. Before I lost the weight, I used to wonder if people could take me seriously. Jorge helped me understand that I was hiding myself behind the weight. Thanks to him and the tools I've learned I've been able to take charge of my life, shed the pounds, and gain the confidence I never had before. Today I feel like my outside reflects who I am on the inside. Besides being able to wear smaller sizes, I can now sleep comfortably through the night, when I used to toss and turn because I was uncomfortable in my own skin. Now I rest easy.

THE 100 | Getting Back to Balance

Mind Over Carb-Madness

In the interest of full disclosure, I must say that, starting any diet, including the one in this book, will have its challenges. Any change we make to our food plans after we've been eating a certain way will take some adjustment. When you alter your pattern of eating to go back to your roots and eat more of a modern-day hunter-gatherer style of diet, which is what I suggest you do for long-term weight loss and health, you will have some struggles. It takes time for you to break the carb-craving cycle, but I promise that on The 100™ you will adjust quickly, and in about a week most of my clients report that cravings have been eliminated. Plus, knowing that you are putting your body back in balance is empowering. Most important, unlike traditional calorie-restrictive, low-fat diets, you won't feel starved or deprived—and you won't be set up to keep craving the foods that get you fat in the first place.

Remember when we talked about that sub sandwich on page 52? This scenario also relates to hunger and cravings. So, imagine you're in line again thinking about your sub, but this time you notice a yummy looking chocolate chip cookie on the counter—research shows that by simply contemplating carbohydrates and sweet foods spikes your insulin dramatically, and it also triggers the reward center of your brain—the same brain regions that are stimulated when an addict uses cocaine or heroin. Whenever an insulin spike occurs, the message it is sending to your cells is "get ready, sugar is on its way, so everyone else get inside your cells," particularly fat molecules, and this chain of events makes you feel the pangs of hunger even more severely.

Insulin also affects the perception of taste: The higher the carbohydrate in the meal or the more sweet the food, the higher your blood sugar, which in turn causes the higher the rise in insulin, and the better the food tastes. If you've been eating a high Sugar Calorie diet for a long time, you predispose your body to store even greater amounts of fat in fat cells, and more protein in muscle cells. Your body has become habituated to this way of being, and won't use fat for fuel because it, your body, has the expectation that more carbs are always coming. This way of eating sets up a strong carb memory that your body adapts to, and this adaptation and expectation causes you to be chained to a hamster wheel of craving even more of the main foods that are making you fat. **It's a horror show of a merry-go-round because the foods that make you fat, also make you crave the foods that make you fat.**

When you eat a diet that is more in line with who and what you are as a biological animal who is evolved to eat high percentages of protein and fats,

JORGE: We are programmed to love sugar. So it is not necessarily our fault genetically, biologically. Right, Gary?

GARY: It is not even a question of whether—I have a bite and I don't think about it. It is my fault and I want more. I just want more. My wife can order dessert, have two bites and push it aside. Then I will take one bite of hers and that dessert starts talking to me. I suspect a lot of overweight, obese people are like this. A lot of thin people too. It is like you—I am sitting here having this dialogue with this dessert sitting on the plate and it is like I can't get the waitress to take it away. I'm in trouble and I end up eating it.

JORGE: It is what we all do. It is normal. It is kind of the human condition.

GARY: Yeah, so it is not a question of I can't eat in moderation. It's the same way I used to be as a smoker. I am a journalist. Smoking was an occupational thing. You can't smoke in moderation. I don't try to smoke in moderation. The same way with alcohol as AA says with Alcoholics Anonymous— once an alcoholic you are always an alcoholic. You don't try to drink in moderation. You realize that you are going to go down the slippery slope. That is at least the way I was with sweets. It is just easier not to do it. And I don't find that suddenly I am having dessert four nights a week again. This happened to me once 10 years ago. A lot of scientists don't like when anecdotal evidence gets into a discussion of science. You may be different than everyone else. I may be different from everyone else. But simultaneously our nutrition is something you can expand upon yourself. If you are naturally lean—my brother was naturally lean and an endurance athlete, I am not—their advice on obesity really isn't all that meaningful. They can read the textbooks. Until you have had a weight problem then you can experiment with what works and what doesn't. You can figure out what carbs your body can tolerate.

and minimal amounts of Sugar Calories (we'll really break this down in the next section) your body starts burning the fat it was hanging on to, you never feel hungry because the foods you eat are slow to digest and keep you full, and since you aren't spiking insulin when you eat this way, you don't sabotage yourself by feeling overly hungry or having carb and sugar cravings.

Evolution-Based Eating for the Modern Human

The solution to all of this is to accept a shift in perception back to a more evolutionary-friendly way of eating, but one that cooperatively coexists with contemporary life. That is just what the The 100™ is designed to do. To match how we are biologically wired to eat, while still taking into account the demands of today's lifestyles, we have to first remember what we discussed in the previous chapter—that for 99.5 percent of our history, a hundred thousand generations of people, we ate diets of high protein and fat, with some vegetables and very little fruit. The foods we eat today have only been around for a mere 10 generations—not nearly enough to be a natural part of our nutritional requirements. It's sort of like climate change and dinosaurs. When a toxic change to the environment happened to these animals, they couldn't survive—that's what our diets are doing to us. Our modern way of eating is in complete contrast to what our bodies need. The result is a society plagued with ever increasing levels of chronic diseases such as obesity, diabetes, cancer, Alzheimer's, and heart disease. The solution is The 100™, because it is crafted to match your genetic blueprint, while avoiding the necessity of strapping on a bow and arrow and heading out into the wild to hunt and forage for food.

We humans are animals—mammals at that—and like any animal on this planet, we are designed to digest a certain diet, just like lions, and tigers, and bears—oh my. Unfortunately most of us eat an unnatural diet, and in response our body sends out alarm signals that cause us to consistently store way too much of our fuel as fat—over time, we are becoming endangered.

When it comes to maintaining a healthy body weight, we need to be able to use the energy we consume from our diets to fuel our bodies appropriately. It helps to think of your pet dog or cat. It's possible to feed your animals a diet formulated to meet their canine or feline needs without providing them with live rabbits or birds for food—even though that's what they were genetically designed to eat. We need to view ourselves in the same light—the answer is in getting back to this biologically, genetically friendly way of eating, without requiring unrealistic, overly restrictive, hard to meet, and out-of-date diets.

When it comes to research on carbohydrate-restricted diets, the findings are promising. In a 2003 study published in the *Journal of Clinical Endocrinology & Metabolism,* University of Cincinnati researchers had 42 obese women follow either an unrestricted (calorie-wise) low-carbohydrate diet, or a calorie-restricted low-fat diet for six months. This is the longest randomized control trial (the gold standard) on record that compares low-carb eating to calorie-restricted diets. Women on both diets reduced calorie consumption even though they weren't required to on the low-carbohydrate diet. The researchers speculated that this might have been due to the satiating effects of the fat and protein in the low-carb group. At the end of the trial, the women in the low-carb group lost more weight than the calorie-restricted group (18.7 pounds vs. 8.6 pounds), and body fat (10.6 pounds vs. 4.4 pounds), and there were no increased signs of heart disease risks in either group. The low-carbohydrate women consumed more than 50 percent of their diet in fat and 20 percent in saturated fat, while the calorie-restricted group consumed 30 percent of their calories from fat. Neither group showed any increase in blood fats (cholesterol).

In another study, published in the *New England Journal of Medicine,* a team of researchers from Philadelphia, Pennsylvania, made up of cardiologists, endocrinologists, and medical experts, had 132 severely obese men and women follow either a low-carbohydrate or a low-fat diet for six months. Nearly 40 percent of these subjects also had diabetes, and more than 40 percent had been diagnosed with metabolic syndrome (for more on metabolic syndrome,

JORGE: With all the research that you have gathered and studied, and really looked at in depth, what do you think is the solution to the obesity epidemic?

GARY: I tell you the solution is getting rid of the sugar, and getting rid of the refined grains. A lot of people will lose a lot of weight. Some people remain obese, but we will turn back this tide. We won't pass it on to our next generation. This gets passed on both genetically and what is called epigenetically from mother to child in the womb, technically called the intrauterine environment. It arguably gets worse every generation. We have more obese mothers. More diabetic mothers. More gestationally diabetic mothers. That means when they become pregnant they become diabetic. In the 1960s, when women got pregnant they were supposed to gain 20 pounds, this was a supposedly a reasonable weight gain. My wife's generation, some of her friends gained 40, 50, 60 pounds when they were pregnant. This works to create children who are predisposed to obesity and diabetes—they need to be born lean. Otherwise, babies will grow into these problems in middle age. Just from what happened to them in the womb.

The way to turn back is to get rid of sugar first, refined grains, starches second. Then arguably you are eating high-fat diets, despite the advice we have been given. Eat fish and meat. You want the fat in the diet. If you look at carnivores. If you look at hunter-gatherer populations, they ate the fattest part of the animals. They ate the fattest animals. They didn't go for the lean. Lean meat was—like lions leave the lean meat for the hyenas and the vultures. They don't want it. They want the fatty organs.

JORGE: For those who want to lose weight, how can you reassure us that fat in the diet is okay, healthy even? People are so scared of fat. There are certain fats, and I'm sure you would agree, such as hydrogenated oils that are man-made fats, that aren't healthy. Give us the quick one minute on what fats to definitely avoid. And what are the fats that we embrace? And how do we get over this issue that they make us fat or cause heart disease?

GARY: Again, I am a believer—the one thing I really agree with Michael Pollan, is that we should eat real food. If you are eating food. You are not eating processed food, you are not eating things that come in boxers, wrappers, cans, you are going to basically get healthy fats.

see page 66). The low-carb diet restricted carbohydrates per day with no restrictions on fat, while the low-fat diet restricted calories enough per person to equal a 500-calorie deficit per day (this given the magical 3,500 calorie deficit a week that is supposed to equal one pound of weight loss per week), plus the low-fat group restricted fat to 30 percent of calories or less. Again, the results found that the low-carbohydrate diet was the winner with people in that group losing more weight than the low-fat group (12.8 pounds vs. 4.2 pounds). The carbohydrate-restricted group also lowered triglyceride levels (the heart damaging and fat producing fats) five times as much as the calorie-restricted group did (20 percent vs. 4 percent), and the low-carb group doubled their level of insulin sensitivity compared to the calorie-restricted group (6 percent vs. 3 percent).

One thing that is discussed by investigators who study carbohydrate-restricted diets is lack of the hunger, weakness, and depression that is reported by people following calorie-restricted diets as discussed earlier in this chapter. In the next section and the following chapters of this book, you'll see how I've designed The 100™ to work in harmony with the way our human bodies are made to eat naturally, and also how The 100™ is set up to work in the real world. As I mentioned above, this is not an extreme Paleo-style diet that will have you foraging in the forest for nuts and seeds. You can eat real foods that are available at your local grocery store.

THE
100 | Conclusion

Recovering alcoholics have a saying: "It's the first drink that gets you drunk," which seems as crazy as saying, "It's the first soda that will get you fat," until you realize that the first drink does chemically alter an alcoholic's brain and body so that he can no longer switch off the desire to drink. Sugar Calories (all carbohydrates), as we've discussed in this chapter, act in just the same way. As soon as you eat that donut or drink that soda, insulin floods your body telling you that you want more. Getting your body back into balance takes commitment and perseverance, but it doesn't have to be difficult, especially with all the tools you now have at your disposal.

You now know how insulin, carbs, and fat work in the body and can reverse your diet to more effectively control weight gain. You know that by reducing the amounts of Sugar Calories you'll not only help yourself to become healthier, you can help generations to come to be fat burners instead of fat loaders.

Congratulations! You now have all the information you need to take action. In the next chapters, we'll get into the specifics of how you'll eat to maximize your weight loss without ever feeling hungry or deprived.

PART TWO

How It Works

"Calories (noun): Tiny creatures that live in your closet and sew your clothes a little bit tighter every night."

The premise is shockingly simple. By simply consuming no more than 100 Sugar Calories per day, you can drop up to 18 pounds in the first two weeks. Here's where we get into the details of how it all works, but before I do that, I want to state my diet philosophy to you clearly.

There are so many terms thrown around about different types of diets—low fat, low carb, carb restricted, Paleo diets, and low glycemic index diets—that it's hard to know what's meant by each of these and where my diet philosophy falls. Let me explain.

Low-fat diets we discussed in the previous chapter—these diets don't work because they promote the foods that cause fat storage and hunger—namely, carbohydrates. New research from Harvard University also shows that these diets dramatically lower your body's calorie burning ability by about 300 calories on a daily basis.

Low carb is a term thrown around a lot, and I include myself in this, but low-carb diets can mean a variety of different things. In the Paleo and Atkins diets, low carb means practically no carbs at all. These diets are made up mostly of meats, some fats, and green vegetables, and while these diets can produce dramatic results, they aren't the healthiest or the most practical plans to follow. The Harvard research mentioned above found that these diets actually increase your ability to burn calories by more than 300 calories per day (a positive), but the trade off isn't worth it because these types of diets also also spike dangerous markers for heart disease (a negative).

Low glycemic index diets These diets are technically low carb because they maximize foods that are low on the glycemic index (an index that ranks foods by their blood-sugar–spiking ability), but still includes grains and some sugars. The same new research from Harvard mentioned above shows that this diet is successful at revving up your daily calorie burn by about 150 calories without spiking heart disease markers. The problem with many of these plans is that they still include carbohydrate levels (Sugar Calories) that slow or halt weight loss effects.

So where does my philosophy fit in? The 100™ is not a low-carb diet or a low-glycemic index diet—rather it is a blend of the best of both worlds. The 100™ does limit your sugar and carb intake naturally by limiting Sugar Calories, which you'll learn about on the next pages; more so than most low glycemic diets, but not to the extremes that the low-carb diets do. The 100™ is a diet that will increase your body's metabolism (your calorie burning engine), speed up weight loss, improve your health, and keep you feeling satisfied (never deprived) so the weight stays off long-term.

In the next chapter, I'll explain the concept behind the Sugar Calories and The 100™ Plan. Then it's time to get started on your weight loss journey, and in chapter 4, I'll get you started with a full four week program that will help you lose up to 18 pounds in the first two weeks. Afterward you can expect to lose 1 to 4 pounds each week consistently. These menus focus on nutritious foods and minimize the Sugar Calories for the fastest, most effective weight loss ever.

> "The 100™ is not a low-carb diet or a low glycemic index diet—rather it is a blend of the best of both worlds."

"I DID IT!"

NICOLE

VITAL STATS

AGE: 40   **HEIGHT:** 5' 1"   **WEIGHT LOST:** 30 pounds

MY BEST STRATEGY: Track it. I keep a chart of everything I eat. It helps me stay conscious about what I'm putting in my mouth and helps me to make better choices because I know I'm accountable. Jorge was my "aha!" moment. His food rules made me aware of a truth I'd been ignoring—I ate way too much sugar that was hidden away in beverages and other foods. Before that, I had been truly blind to the fact that I had an unhealthy diet. I used to blame my family and my genes for my weight. I'd also make excuses about being overstressed and having bad luck. This allowed me to shirk responsibility and pretend like I was just powerless to being overweight. I used to feel so sluggish in the mornings and at night. Now that I eat the Jorge way, I have more energy than I know what to do with. Plus, I feel confident and good about my body. I am inspired every day.

3

Understanding Sugar Calories

I've been on a constant diet for the last two
decades. I've lost a total of 789 pounds. By
all accounts, I should be hanging from a
charm bracelet.

—ERMA BOMBECK

If you are not sitting down, please take a seat and prepare yourself. I am about to release the most controversial yet breakthrough point of discussion of this entire book. In the last few chapters you have discovered that diets fail, the calories-in/calories-out philosophy is inaccurate and has no bearing on lasting weight loss or nutrition. Low (or no) carb programs like Atkins and Paleo diets are unsustainable and not enjoyable for long-term success. The reason that these diets have let so many down in the past is because they do not hold the specific key to weight loss—a fundamental truth that the world has been ignoring:

All carbohydrates are actually structured as sugars molecularly.

When speaking to many around the world on the subject of weight management, many women have told me that they are aware that sugar is bad, and you may even be nodding your head and saying, "Of course it is, I know that," but it may surprise you—as it does most of my clients—to learn that all carbohydrates are made up of chains of sugars, and in your body they affect your insulin just like sugar. And left unchecked—all these carbohydrates can cause weight gain. I am not saying all carbohydrates and sugars are completely equal, I am saying that molecularly they have the same base structure. And both sugars and carbohydrates have controls on the master gauge of insulin. So from now on I want you to understand that *when I say Sugar Calories I mean all carbohydrates including starchy vegetables, breads, grains, crackers, cookies, donuts, sugars, honey, juices, sodas, and so on.*

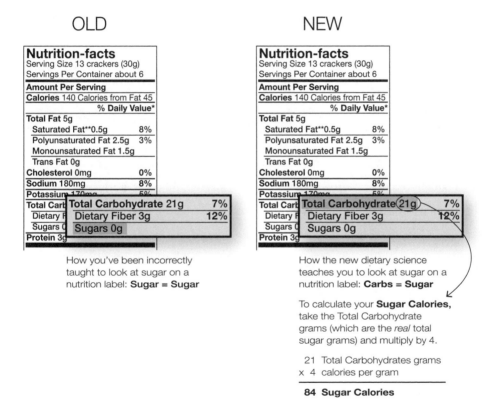

OLD

How you've been incorrectly taught to look at sugar on a nutrition label: **Sugar = Sugar**

NEW

How the new dietary science teaches you to look at sugar on a nutrition label: **Carbs = Sugar**

To calculate your **Sugar Calories,** take the Total Carbohydrate grams (which are the *real* total sugar grams) and multiply by 4.

21 Total Carbohydrates grams
x 4 calories per gram
_____
84 Sugar Calories

Let me say it plainly: From this point forward I want you to look at that loaf of bread sitting in your kitchen as a loaf of sugar, the crackers and pasta in your cupboard—also sugar, the "energy" bars packed away in your car—little bars of sugar.

The beauty of The 100™ is that you still get to have sugar! And it's simple, you get 100 Sugar Calories, and the rest of the foods you will eat fall under the Freebie categories. These Freebies don't have to be tracked because they don't spike insulin, and won't cause weight gain. The 100 Sugar Calories come from ideally nutritious sources, but gives you the freedom to choose foods that may not be considered "diet food" when you really want them. Imagine, eating out, special occasions, or a simple evening with some chocolate and wine, all good things to make life enjoyable. For my clients, it's surprising that they can effortlessly lose weight while still getting to have real life, modern-day foods, and never feel hungry.

The foods to focus on: Where it gets fun is you actually get to have lots of nutritious sugar from wonderful sources. Lets take a look at a sample meal that falls under the Freebie foods. For a full list of foods on Freebie list, turn to The 100™ Food Lists in chapter 8.

For a moment, be very quiet and see if you cannot hear the crackling of diced bacon in a hot cast iron skillet, the aroma fills the room and then it is time to add quartered brussel sprouts to the sizzling bacon. Caramelizing the edges of the sprouts as you gently move the pan back and forth, you watch them break down and get soft to the fork's touch, you add a pinch of salt as they fall to your plate next to a garlic baked chicken breast. These are just a couple of the freebie foods you can enjoy.

As I take a step back and regroup from this kitchen experience, I want you to know that those brussel sprouts do contain sugar, that's right, another shocker I am sure. In fact, a half cup contains 148 sugar calories. However, and this is important, only sugars that come from starchy vegetables, legumes and grains (refined and whole) are categorized under the Sugar Calories you count. Meaning that those brussel sprouts are OK! All other categories do not count. The reason is simple: the amount of Sugar Calories, divided by the volume, multiplied by the fiber content would not be enough to cause a rise in insulin. Plus eating an abundant source of vegetables will help you reach the

American Heart Association's recommendation of 25 to 30 grams of fiber per day as well as provide you essential nutrients and vitamins. Okay, that little calculation might not be so easy for you to do on each and every food you eat, but that's why I've done the work for you—with my menus, food lists, and guidelines, you won't need to worry about any messy calculations.

I could write a whole book based on why vegetables, especially fresh, are so good for your body long term. Other items that are on the "Freebie" list are good fats and protein such as olive oil, chicken breast, etc. . . . Please do not think that I am recommending anybody eat more of these types of foods than is necessary. You will notice some portion recommendations in the next chapter for your 4 week menus that will guide you, and while you won't have to think much about how to eat because I've done the work for you, here are a few pointers.

Water. From the research I have done the simple answer to "How much water?" is have water when you are thirsty, and don't drink it when you are not. Oftentimes when you are craving something or jonesing for a soda, your body is really asking to be hydrated. If you are exercising or working out, that is a great time to keep some water on hand. My rule of thumb is to keep a (bpa free) water bottle on hand, and don't be afraid to take a sip every once in a while.

Portions. I went out to breakfast one day and saw the oddest thing. A man ordered 12 strips of bacon and 8 scrambled eggs. Shocked his friend asked what he was doing and he said he was "Paleo" and this was in accordance with his diet. Wow! Here is the point: 12 strips of bacon are not good for you; really, excess of anything is not good for you. Fortunately the foods on the Freebie list are hard to overeat, and I have not heard of anybody overdosing on broccoli. But the saying "everything in moderation" does apply here. So here are my official guidelines for a typical meal. Note: You can always do less than the maximum here, and not eating when you are not hungry has been shown to be good for you. So, if you aren't in the mood for breakfast, you have my permission to skip it.

BUT WHAT ABOUT BREAKFAST?

"It's the most important meal of the day," right? Not necessarily, according to new research, as well as old logic. It's understandable that most of us believe this because it's part of conventional wisdom—we've read about it, or heard it from nutritionists and doctors—but that isn't accurate advice. I know clients who actually hide the fact that they skip breakfast because they feel ashamed of it. Well, there's no need. Actually, research from the *British Journal of Nutrition* shows that skipping breakfast, while it does lead to slightly more intake of food during the rest of the day, still results in less eating overall at the end of the day. There's also some evidence that this approach lowers blood sugar and causes an increase in insulin sensitivity. Think about the name "breakfast." It actually is a phrase that defines the time of day you decide to "break" your "fast." This means that your "breaking of the fast," or your breakfast can be any time of day you want. Some people find that if they eat from 11 a.m. to 8 p.m., instead of from 6 a.m. to 7 p.m., that they eat less overall as well. I'm not suggesting that you do this every day, but once or twice a week is a great strategy if it fits your schedule.

I suggest that you begin by trying a delayed breakfast one day out of your week. After you've done this for a few weeks and decided that it is something that works for you, you can then increase to two days a week.

What to do: Have your breakfast at 11 a.m. and your last meal of the day by 8 p.m. on the day of your morning fast. Make sure you drink plenty of water, and don't use this method on consecutive days. Instead separate your days: delay breakfast on Tuesday, and then have an early breakfast on Wednesday, do a morning fast again on Thursday.

By skipping the traditional breakfast—as discussed earlier—you won't eat as much during the rest of the day—a sneaky, but effective dieting plan. Here's how I do it—a late breakfast, usually a couple scrambled eggs and some bacon, and then an early dinner, usually fish and veggies. In addition, I drink plenty of calorie free beverages: coffee, tea, water.

Breaking the Fast On the day and time of your break-fast the goal is to act as if your fast never happened. Eat The 100™ way, and enjoy yourself.

Exercise The benefits of fasting do appear to be increased for people who include strength training two to three times a week. This helps with the rate of fat burn, weight loss, and maintaining muscle mass—please see page 198 for the workout I included.

- Ask yourself if you are actually hungry for your next bite.

- If you feel full, you have overeaten.

- Freebie Veggies—Half your plate maximum (unless you have had your entire plate and are actually hungry, feel free to have another serving for this meal).

- Freebie Protein—Deck of cards or 3 oz. (for men or those who are looking to build muscle you may go up to 6 oz.).

- Freebie Fats—Bottle cap or 1 oz. (this amount can vary up and down slightly, but try to stick to this range.)

- Sugar Calories—My recommendation is not to have any given meal reach the full 100 Sugar Calories but rather try to distribute them throughout the day. You may feel that this meal needed a condiment that contains Sugar Calories or perhaps a slice of whole grain toast would be best. The good part is that when making your own meals you get to make the choice. Typically, I advise my clients to reserve their Sugar Calories for the end of the day to make sure they do not accidentally go over.

These are just some quick suggestions. In the next chapter, you'll get everything you need for your next four weeks of eating and losing weight The 100™ way.

JORGE: We think fat makes us fat. Does fat not make us fat, Gary?

GARY: No. No. Fat doesn't make you fat.

JORGE: Take a minute on that.

GARY: If we eat a high-fat diet, that means a high saturated fat diet, then basically your body runs the way it is supposed to run. It is that simple. One of the things I learned from studying medicine, medical research the last 25 years, is that we tend to oversimplify things—the old thinking, eating fat makes us fat is incorrect. What matters is what your body does with carbohydrates because carbohydrates stimulate insulin, which locks fat away in the fat tissue. The fat does get stored in your fat tissue first. But it is the carbohydrates that keep the fat in there. So the carbs are the problem even if the first thing you store is fat. If you don't have carbs your body will put the fat in the fat tissue, but then it will let it out of the fat tissue and burn it for fuel, which is what it is supposed to do.

You think of it like money—say most of us when we go to the ATM and we have money you know like say money for the week, 300 dollars. We put it in our wallet. And then everywhere we go we dole it out and at the end of the week we get more. That is how our fat tissues should work. Like that wallet. Not like some long-term savings account in the bank. Where you put it in and you accumulate for your kids' college education and then they go to college and it is locked away, you forgot the combination or the account number.

JORGE: Carbohydrates cause fat to lock in.

GARY: They do. So then you keep putting money into the wallet but you can't get it out. The wallet gets fatter and fatter.

Now you are ready to start The 100™. On the next pages, you'll find your four week menu, filled with delicious ideas and options. The 100 Sugar Calories have been calculated for you, so your eating will be a breeze.

" I DID IT! "

NATALIE

VITAL STATS

AGE: 52   **HEIGHT:** 5' 7"   **WEIGHT LOST:** 15 pounds

BEST STRATEGY: Be prepared for a sweet tooth. I carry stevia packets with me in my purse. Before I found Jorge, I had a big fat belly—I hated the way I looked in clothes and I always felt worn out and tired. I hated that I couldn't keep up with my four kids, and I know I have grandkids in my future, and I couldn't stand the idea of not being around for them. I love eating this way because it is so easy to do—there's so little to track and think about—I can just enjoy my life. I have plenty of energy now that the excess weight is gone, and I love to exercise all the time. This is the way I will eat for the rest of my life.

Your Four Week Plan

Most of what we need to know about how
to eat we already know, or once did until
we allowed the nutrition experts and the
advertisers to shake our confidence in
common sense, tradition, the testimony of
our senses, and the wisdom of our mothers
and grandmothers.

—MICHAEL POLLAN, FOOD EXPERT AND

AUTHOR OF *IN DEFENSE OF FOOD.*

It's time to get started! I have made it super simple by providing you with
four weeks of done-for-you menus. The following menus maximize the
healthy freebies, and focus on the best of the Sugar Calories (the healthiest of
carbs as described in chapter 8), so that your insulin will stay at minimum levels,
which will allow your fat cells to be activated to release the most amount of fat
possible.

Yes, you can drop up to 18 pounds in the first two weeks on The 100™, just understand that not all of that weight will come directly from fat. Only about five or six pounds will be burned from your fat stores. Where will the rest of the weight come from? The rest is what I like to call "false fat," which is simply trapped waste matter in your body. I know it is unpleasant to imagine this buildup in your body, but the good news is you are flushing these toxins from your system in just one week! Plus, it is slimming. A lot of what may be giving you a bloated feeling is built-up waste in your intestines, the result of a lack of good carbohydrates in your daily eating plan. The fiber that comes from the Freebies list in chapter 8 is critical for removing this kind of waste from your body; eating a diet of highly refined, easily digestible, and processed carbs and sugars fails to sweep out your intestines. You will experience the weight loss that's right for you (see the chart on the next page). Your results will be dramatic, and you will look and feel fantastic and renewed.

When following the four week plan I have **two different paths** you can take. One path gives total freedom to enjoy different meals as you choose, and the other is pure simplicity. Feel free to choose one of the following options:

Option 1: Follow the 1 Menu

I recommend this option for those who really like automation and the freedom to choose what you want to eat. Simply use The 1 Menu for seven days, which is the most affordable option, or mix and match from the options page when you would like. You get to decide between the meals. To create a meal planner and shopping list for the week, grab a piece of paper and plot out your week between The 1 Menu and your Options. When finished, add up all the foods and you've got yourself a shopping list.

Or

Option 2: Follow My Meal Planner

I recommend this option for busy people who are looking for a guaranteed plan. Simply follow each meal in the Meal Planner as recommended. Use the shopping list to stock up for the week. Some of my most successful clients prepare as much of the food ahead of time to make their meals effortless. Done-for-you, easy weight control.

Your Goal Total	Each Week
Lose 30 to 60 pounds	6 to 9 pounds
Lose 10 to 29 pounds	4 to 6 pounds
Lose 3 to 9 pounds	1 to 4 pounds

The 1 Menu

Breakfast: 1 Skinny Muffin with butter, served with coffee with half-and-half
(see Skinny Muffin recipe on page 139)
(0 SUGAR CALORIES, not 353 calories)

Snack: 1 string cheese stick
(0 SUGAR CALORIES, not 80 calories)

Lunch: 2 cups shredded Romaine lettuce tossed in 2 Tbsp. Caesar dressing and
topped with 5 grilled shrimp and 1 Tbsp. grated Parmesan cheese
(4 SUGAR CALORIES, not 224 calories)

Snack: 1 slice deli turkey and 1 slice American cheese
(0 SUGAR CALORIES, not 101 calories)

Dinner: 1 grilled flank steak, cut intro strips, tossed with 2 cups spinach, 5 cherry
tomatoes, and olive oil/red wine vinegar dressing
(0 SUGAR CALORIES, not 306 calories)

Treat: Up to 2 glasses red wine
(29 SUGAR CALORIES, not 437 Calories)

TOTAL: 33 SUGAR CALORIES, not 1501 Calories

Options

Breakfast: 2 eggs scrambled with ¼ cup red bell pepper, ½ cup spinach, ½ cup grated cheddar cheese, served with a side of 2 strips bacon and coffee with half-and-half
(0 SUGAR CALORIES, not 530 Calories)

Lunch: ½ head iceberg lettuce topped with 2 strips chopped cooked bacon, 1 chopped hard-boiled egg, 2 Tbsp. chopped tomatoes, 2 Tbsp. chopped cucumbers, 2 Tbsp. blue cheese crumbles, and 2 Tbsp. blue cheese dressing
(6 SUGAR CALORIES, not 419 Calories)

Tuna salad made of 1 can tuna, 2 Tbsp. mayonnaise and 1 Tbsp. lime juice, served on 2 Romaine leaf halves
(0 SUGAR CALORIES, not 647 Calories)

Dinner: 1 chicken breast rubbed with 1 Tbsp. Dijon mustard and 1 tsp. black pepper, panfried in 1 Tbsp. olive oil, served with a side salad of 1 cup spinach, 2 Tbsp. chopped red pepper, 2 Tbsp. chopped green onion, and ¼ cup chopped zucchini, drizzled with olive oil and vinegar for dressing
(0 SUGAR CALORIES, not 397 Calories)

1 orange roughy fillet dipped in 1 beaten egg, then dipped in Parmesan cheese, cooked in 1 Tbsp. olive oil for 3–4 minutes on each side, served with a side of ½ cup cooked green beans seasoned with salt and pepper
(0 SUGAR CALORIES, not 349 Calories)

Snacks: ¼ cup walnuts
(0 SUGAR CALORIES, not 191 Calories)

1 hard-boiled egg
(0 SUGAR CALORIES, not 80 Calories)

Meal Planner: **MONDAY**

Breakfast

1 Skinny Muffin with butter, served with coffee with half-and-half (see Skinny Muffin recipe on page 139)

(0 SUGAR CALORIES, not 353 Calories)

Snack

1 string cheese stick

(0 SUGAR CALORIES, not 80 Calories)

Lunch

2 cups shredded Romaine lettuce tossed in 2 Tbsp. Caesar dressing and topped with 5 grilled shrimp, and 1 Tbsp. grated Parmesan cheese

(4 SUGAR CALORIES, not 224 Calories)

Snack

1 slice deli turkey & 1 slice American cheese

(0 SUGAR CALORIES, not 101 Calories)

Dinner

1 grilled flank steak, cut intro strips, tossed with 2 cups spinach, 5 cherry tomatoes, and olive oil/red wine vinegar dressing

(0 SUGAR CALORIES, not 306 calories)

Treat

Up to 2 glasses red wine

(29 SUGAR CALORIES, not 437 Calories)

TOTAL 33 SUGAR CALORIES, not 1501 calories

Meal Planner: **TUESDAY**

Breakfast

2 eggs scrambled with ¼ cup red bell pepper, ½ cup spinach, ½ cup grated cheddar cheese, served with a side of 2 strips bacon and coffee with half-and-half

(0 SUGAR CALORIES, not 530 Calories)

Snack

¼ cup walnuts

(0 SUGAR CALORIES, not 191 Calories)

Lunch

½ head iceberg lettuce topped with 2 strips chopped cooked bacon, 1 chopped hard-boiled egg, 2 Tbsp. chopped tomatoes, 2 Tbsp. chopped cucumbers, 2 Tbsp. blue cheese crumbles, and 2 Tbsp. blue cheese dressing

(6 SUGAR CALORIES, not 419 Calories)

Snack

1 hard-boiled egg

(0 SUGAR CALORIES, not 80 Calories)

Dinner

1 chicken breast rubbed with 1 Tbsp. Dijon mustard and 1 tsp. black pepper, panfried in 1 Tbsp. olive oil, served with a side salad of 1 cup spinach, 2 Tbsp. chopped red pepper, 2 Tbsp. chopped green onion, and ¼ cup chopped zucchini, drizzled with olive oil and vinegar for dressing

(0 SUGAR CALORIES, not 397 Calories)

Treat

Up to 2 glasses red wine

(29 SUGAR CALORIES, not 437 Calories)

TOTAL 35 SUGAR CALORIES, not 2054 Calories

Meal Planner: WEDNESDAY

Breakfast

1 Skinny Muffin with butter, served with coffee with half-and-half (see Skinny Muffin recipe on page 139)

(0 SUGAR CALORIES, not 353 Calories)

Snack

1 string cheese stick

(0 SUGAR CALORIES, not 80 Calories)

Lunch

Tuna salad made of 1 can tuna, 2 Tbsp. mayonnaise and 1 Tbsp. lime juice, served on 2 Romaine leaf halves

(0 SUGAR CALORIES, not 647 Calories)

Snack

1 slice deli turkey & 1 slice American cheese

(0 SUGAR CALORIES, not 101 Calories)

Dinner

1 orange roughy fillet dipped in 1 beaten egg, then dipped in Parmesan cheese, cooked in 1 Tbsp. olive oil for 3–4 minutes on each side, served with a side of ½ cup cooked green beans seasoned with salt and pepper

(0 SUGAR CALORIES, not 349 Calories)

Treat

Up to 2 glasses red wine

(29 SUGAR CALORIES, not 437 Calories)

TOTAL 29 SUGAR CALORIES, not 1967 Calories

Meal Planner: **THURSDAY**

Breakfast

2 eggs scrambled with ¼ cup red bell pepper, ½ cup spinach, ½ cup grated cheddar cheese, served with a side of 2 strips bacon and coffee with half-and-half

(0 SUGAR CALORIES, not 530 Calories)

Snack

¼ cup walnuts

(0 SUGAR CALORIES, not 191 Calories)

Lunch

2 cups shredded Romaine lettuce tossed in 2 Tbsp. Caesar dressing and topped with 5 grilled shrimp, and 1 Tbsp. grated Parmesan cheese

(4 SUGAR CALORIES, not 224 Calories)

Snack

1 hard-boiled egg

(0 SUGAR CALORIES, not 80 Calories)

Dinner

1 grilled flank steak, cut intro strips, tossed with 2 cups spinach, 5 cherry tomatoes, and olive oil/red wine vinegar dressing

(0 SUGAR CALORIES, not 306 Calories)

Treat

Up to 2 glasses red wine

(29 SUGAR CALORIES, not 437 Calories)

TOTAL 33 SUGAR CALORIES, not 1768 Calories

Meal Planner: **FRIDAY**

Breakfast

1 Skinny Muffin with butter, served with coffee with half-and-half (see Skinny Muffin recipe on page 139)

(0 SUGAR CALORIES, not 353 Calories)

Snack

1 string cheese stick

(0 SUGAR CALORIES, not 80 Calories)

Lunch

½ head iceberg lettuce topped with 2 strips chopped cooked bacon, 1 chopped hard-boiled egg, 2 Tbsp. chopped tomatoes, 2 Tbsp. chopped cucumbers, 2 Tbsp. blue cheese crumbles, and 2 Tbsp. blue cheese dressing

(6 SUGAR CALORIES, not 419 Calories)

Snack

1 slice deli turkey & 1 slice American cheese

(0 SUGAR CALORIES, not 101 Calories)

Dinner

1 chicken breast rubbed with 1 Tbsp. Dijon mustard and 1 tsp. black pepper, panfried in 1 Tbsp. olive oil, served with a side salad of 1 cup spinach, 2 Tbsp. chopped red pepper, 2 Tbsp. chopped green onion, and ¼ cup chopped zucchini, drizzled with olive oil and vinegar for dressing

(0 SUGAR CALORIES, not 397 Calories)

Treat

Up to 2 glasses red wine

(29 SUGAR CALORIES, not 437 Calories)

TOTAL 38 SUGAR CALORIES, not 1787 Calories

Meal Planner: **SATURDAY**

Breakfast

2 eggs scrambled with ¼ cup red bell pepper, ½ cup spinach, ½ cup grated cheddar cheese, served with a side of 2 strips bacon and coffee with half-and-half

(0 SUGAR CALORIES, not 530 Calories)

Snack

¼ cup walnuts

(0 SUGAR CALORIES, not 191 Calories)

Lunch

Tuna salad made of 1 can tuna, 2 Tbsp. mayonnaise and 1 Tbsp. lime juice, served on 2 Romaine leaf halves

(0 SUGAR CALORIES, not 647 Calories)

Snack

1 hard-boiled egg

(0 SUGAR CALORIES, not 80 Calories)

Dinner

1 orange roughy fillet dipped in 1 beaten egg, then dipped in Parmesan cheese, cooked in 1 Tbsp. olive oil for 3–4 minutes on each side, served with a side of ½ cup cooked green beans seasoned with salt and pepper

(0 SUGAR CALORIES, not 349 Calories)

Treat

Up to 2 glasses red wine

(29 SUGAR CALORIES, not 437 Calories)

TOTAL 29 SUGAR CALORIES, not 2234 Calories

Meal Planner: **SUNDAY**

Breakfast

1 Skinny Muffin with butter, served with coffee with half-and-half (see Skinny Muffin recipe on page 139)

(0 SUGAR CALORIES, not 353 Calories)

Snack

1 string cheese stick

(0 SUGAR CALORIES, not 80 Calories)

Lunch

2 cups shredded Romaine lettuce tossed in 2 Tbsp. Caesar dressing and topped with 5 grilled shrimp, and 1 Tbsp. grated Parmesan cheese

(4 SUGAR CALORIES, not 224 Calories)

Snack

1 slice deli turkey & 1 slice American cheese

(0 SUGAR CALORIES, not 101 Calories)

Dinner

1 grilled flank steak, cut intro strips, tossed with 2 cups spinach, 5 cherry tomatoes, and olive oil/red wine vinegar dressing

(0 SUGAR CALORIES, not 306 Calories)

Treat

Up to 2 glasses red wine

(29 SUGAR CALORIES, not 437 Calories)

TOTAL 33 SUGAR CALORIES, not 1501 Calories

Shopping List

Produce

1 red bell pepper

4 Tbsp. chopped green
    onion

½ cup chopped zucchini

1 cup green beans

1½ heads iceberg lettuce

6 cups shredded
    Romaine lettuce

2 Romaine lettuce leaves

9½ cups spinach

2 Tbsp. lime juice

15 cherry tomatoes

4 Tbsp. chopped tomato

4 Tbsp. chopped
    cucumber

Meat/Fish

10 strips bacon

4 slices deli turkey

15 shrimp

2 cans tuna

2 orange roughy fillets

2 chicken breasts

2 flank steaks

Dairy

half-and-half

butter

17 eggs

4 Tbsp. blue cheese
    crumbles

1½ cups grated cheddar
    cheese

4 string cheese sticks

4 slices American cheese

grated Parmesan cheese

Other

coffee

red wine

red wine vinegar

vinegar

olive oil

salt

pepper

4 Stevia/Truvia packets

8 tsp. cinnamon
    powder

coconut oil

baking powder

1 cup ground flax

4 Tbsp. blue cheese
    dressing

4 Tbsp. mayonnaise

2 Tbsp. Dijon mustard

6 Tbsp. Caesar dressing

¾ cup walnuts

The 1 Menu

Breakfast: 2 eggs, sunny-side up, served over 8 asparagus spears, topped with 1 Tbsp. shaved Parmesan cheese, served with coffee with half-and-half
(0 SUGAR CALORIES, not 148 Calories)

Snack: ¼ cup pumpkin seeds
(0 SUGAR CALORIES, not 71 Calories)

Lunch: Shrimp salad made of 8 cooked baby shrimp mixed with 1 Tbsp. mayo, 2 Tbsp. chopped celery, 1 tsp. lemon juice, 1 tsp. lime juice, and 1 tsp. chopped dill, served on a Romaine lettuce leaf
(0 SUGAR CALORIES, not 151 Calories)

Snack: 3 celery sticks spread with cream cheese
(0 SUGAR CALORIES, not 60 Calories)

Dinner: 1 chicken breast panfried in 1 Tbsp. olive oil, 1 Tbsp. balsamic vinegar, and 2 tsp. garlic, served with a side of 6 asparagus spears and 5 cherry tomatoes that have both been drizzled lightly with balsamic vinegar and cooked in the oven for 10 minutes at 500 degrees, then topped with 8 cubes mozzarella cheese
(12 SUGAR CALORIES, not 311 calories)

Treat: Up to 2 glasses red wine
(29 SUGAR CALORIES, not 437 Calories)

TOTAL: 41 SUGAR CALORIES, not 1178 Calories

Options

Breakfast: 2 eggs beaten with 2 Tbsp. half-and-half, ⅛ tsp. salt, ⅛ tsp. pepper, ¼ cup shredded cheddar cheese, ¼ cup chopped zucchini, ¼ cup chopped red bell pepper, and 1 Tbsp. chopped red onion, divided into 2 muffin tin cups and baked at 350 degrees for about 20 minutes, served with coffee with half-and-half
(0 SUGAR CALORIES, not 330 Calories)

Lunch: 1 turkey breast, cooked and shredded, mixed with 2 Tbsp. chopped green onion, 2 Tbsp. chopped cilantro, 1 Tbsp. lime juice, ¼ avocado, and 2 Tbsp. mayo served on a Romaine leaf
(0 SUGAR CALORIES, not 419 Calories)

2 steak kebabs, each made with 3 (1-inch) cubes grilled steak, 3 slices grilled zucchini, 2 slices grilled eggplant, and 2 slices grilled onion, served with a side salad of 1 cup mixed greens with olive oil, salt, and pepper
(0 SUGAR CALORIES, not 383 Calories)

Dinner: 1 grilled salmon fillet served over 1 cup arugula and topped with ¼ cup sautéed asparagus, ¼ cup sautéed red bell pepper, and ¼ cup sautéed zucchini
(0 SUGAR CALORIES, not 198 Calories)

2 cups shredded Romaine lettuce topped with 1 sliced cooked chicken breast, 5 sliced cherry tomatoes, 2 Tbsp. chopped steamed broccoli, 2 Tbsp. sliced onion, 2 Tbsp. marinara sauce, 2 tsp. dried oregano, 2 tsp. dried basil, 4 slices cooked pepperoni and 2 Tbsp. Parmesan cheese
(8 SUGAR CALORIES, not 403 Calories)

Snacks: ¼ cup chopped raw broccoli dipped in mustard
(0 SUGAR CALORIES, not 15 Calories)

¼ cup pecans
(0 SUGAR CALORIES, not 171 Calories)

Meal Planner: MONDAY

Breakfast

2 eggs, sunny-side up served over 8 asparagus spears, topped with 1 Tbsp. shaved Parmesan cheese, served with coffee with half-and-half

(0 SUGAR CALORIES, not 148 Calories)

Snack

¼ cup pumpkin seeds

(0 SUGAR CALORIES, not 71 Calories)

Lunch

Shrimp salad made of 8 cooked baby shrimp mixed with 1 Tbsp. mayo, 2 Tbsp. chopped celery, 1 tsp. lemon juice, 1 tsp. lime juice, and 1 tsp. chopped dill, served on a Romaine lettuce leaf

(0 SUGAR CALORIES, not 151 Calories)

Snack

3 celery sticks spread with cream cheese

(0 SUGAR CALORIES, not 60 Calories)

Dinner

1 chicken breast panfried in 1 Tbsp. olive oil, 1 Tbsp. balsamic vinegar, and 2 tsp. garlic, served with a side of 6 asparagus spears and 5 cherry tomatoes that have both been drizzled lightly with balsamic vinegar and cooked in the oven for 10 minutes at 500 degrees, then topped with 8 cubes mozzarella cheese

(12 SUGAR CALORIES, not 311 calories)

Treat

Up to 2 glasses red wine

(29 SUGAR CALORIES, not 437 Calories)

TOTAL 41 SUGAR CALORIES, not 1178 Calories

Meal Planner: TUESDAY

Breakfast

2 eggs beaten with 2 Tbsp. half-and-half, ⅛ tsp. salt, ⅛ tsp. pepper, ¼ cup shredded cheddar cheese, ¼ cup chopped zucchini, ¼ cup chopped red bell pepper, and 1 Tbsp. chopped red onion, divided into 2 muffin tin cups and baked at 350 degrees for about 20 minutes, served with coffee with half-and-half

(0 SUGAR CALORIES, not 330 Calories)

Snack

¼ cup chopped raw broccoli dipped in mustard

(0 SUGAR CALORIES, not 15 Calories)

Lunch

1 turkey breast, cooked and shredded, mixed with 2 Tbsp. chopped green onion, 2 Tbsp. chopped cilantro, 1 Tbsp. lime juice, ¼ avocado, and 2 Tbsp. mayo served on a romaine leaf

(0 SUGAR CALORIES, not 419 Calories)

Snack

¼ cup pecans

(0 SUGAR CALORIES, not 171 Calories)

Dinner

1 grilled salmon fillet served over a bed of 1 cup arugula and topped with ¼ cup sautéed asparagus, ¼ cup sautéed red bell pepper, and ¼ cup sautéed zucchini

(0 SUGAR CALORIES, not 198 Calories)

Treat

Up to 2 glasses red wine

(29 SUGAR CALORIES, not 437 Calories)

TOTAL 29 SUGAR CALORIES, not 1570 Calories

Meal Planner: WEDNESDAY

Breakfast

2 eggs, sunny-side up served over 8 asparagus spears, topped with 1 Tbsp. shaved Parmesan cheese, served with coffee with half-and-half

(0 SUGAR CALORIES, not 148 Calories)

Snack

¼ cup pumpkin seeds

(0 SUGAR CALORIES, not 71 Calories)

Lunch

2 steak kebabs, each made with 3 (1-inch) cubes grilled steak, 3 slices grilled zucchini, 2 slices grilled eggplant, and 2 slices grilled onion, served with a side salad of 1 cup mixed greens with olive oil, salt, and pepper

(0 SUGAR CALORIES, not 383 Calories)

Snack

3 celery sticks spread with cream cheese

(0 SUGAR CALORIES, not 60 Calories)

Dinner

2 cups shredded Romaine lettuce topped with 1 sliced cooked chicken breast, 5 sliced cherry tomatoes, 2 Tbsp. chopped steamed broccoli, 2 Tbsp. sliced red onion, 2 Tbsp. marinara sauce, 2 tsp. dried oregano, 2 tsp. dried basil, 4 slices cooked pepperoni and 2 Tbsp. Parmesan cheese

(8 SUGAR CALORIES, not 403 Calories)

Treat

Up to 2 glasses red wine

(29 SUGAR CALORIES, not 437 Calories)

TOTAL 37 SUGAR CALORIES, not 1502 Calories

Meal Planner: THURSDAY

Breakfast

2 eggs beaten with 2 Tbsp. half-and-half, ⅛ tsp. salt, ⅛ tsp. pepper, ¼ cup shredded cheddar cheese, ¼ cup chopped zucchini, ¼ cup chopped red bell pepper, and 1 Tbsp. chopped red onion, divided into 2 muffin tin cups and baked at 350 degrees for about 20 minutes, served with coffee with half-and-half

(0 SUGAR CALORIES, not 330 Calories)

Snack

¼ cup chopped raw broccoli dipped in mustard

(0 SUGAR CALORIES, not 15 Calories)

Lunch

Shrimp salad made of 8 cooked baby shrimp mixed with 1 Tbsp. mayo, 2 Tbsp. chopped celery, 1 tsp. lemon juice, 1 tsp. lime juice, and 1 tsp. chopped dill, served on a Romaine lettuce leaf

(0 SUGAR CALORIES, not 151 Calories)

Snack

¼ cup pecans

(0 SUGAR CALORIES, not 171 Calories)

Dinner

1 chicken breast panfried in 1 Tbsp. olive oil, 1 Tbsp. balsamic vinegar, and 2 tsp. garlic, served with a side of 6 asparagus spears and 5 cherry tomatoes that have both been drizzled lightly with balsamic vinegar and cooked in the oven for 10 minutes at 500 degrees, then topped with 8 cubes mozzarella cheese

(12 SUGAR CALORIES, not 311 calories)

Treat

Up to 2 glasses red wine

(29 SUGAR CALORIES, not 437 Calories)

*TOTAL 41 SUGAR CALORIES, **not 1415 Calories***

Meal Planner: FRIDAY

Breakfast

2 eggs, sunny-side up served over 8 asparagus spears, topped with 1 Tbsp. shaved Parmesan cheese, served with coffee with half-and-half

(0 SUGAR CALORIES, not 148 Calories)

Snack

¼ cup pumpkin seeds

(0 SUGAR CALORIES, not 71 Calories)

Lunch

1 turkey breast, cooked and shredded, mixed with 2 Tbsp. chopped green onion, 2 Tbsp. chopped cilantro, 1 Tbsp. lime juice, ¼ avocado, and 2 Tbsp. mayo served on a Romaine leaf

(0 SUGAR CALORIES, not 419 Calories)

Snack

3 celery sticks spread with cream cheese

(0 SUGAR CALORIES, not 60 Calories)

Dinner

1 grilled salmon fillet served over a bed of 1 cup arugula and topped with ¼ cup sautéed asparagus, ¼ cup sautéed red bell pepper, and ¼ cup sautéed zucchini

(0 SUGAR CALORIES, not 198 Calories)

Treat

Up to 2 glasses red wine

(29 SUGAR CALORIES, not 437 Calories)

TOTAL 29 SUGAR CALORIES, not 1333 Calories

Meal Planner: SATURDAY

Breakfast

2 eggs beaten with 2 Tbsp. half-and-half, ⅛ tsp. salt, ⅛ tsp. pepper, ¼ cup shredded cheddar cheese, ¼ cup chopped zucchini, ¼ cup chopped red bell pepper, and 1 Tbsp. chopped red onion, divided into 2 muffin tin cups and baked at 350 degrees for about 20 minutes, served with coffee with half-and-half

(0 SUGAR CALORIES, not 330 Calories)

Snack

¼ cup chopped raw broccoli dipped in mustard

(0 SUGAR CALORIES, not 15 Calories)

Lunch

2 steak kebabs, each made with 3 (1-inch) cubes grilled steak, 3 slices grilled zucchini, 2 slices grilled eggplant, and 2 slices grilled onion, served with a side salad of 1 cup mixed greens with olive oil, salt, and pepper

(0 SUGAR CALORIES, not 383 Calories)

Snack

¼ cup pecans

(0 SUGAR CALORIES, not 171 Calories)

Dinner

2 cups shredded Romaine lettuce topped with 1 sliced cooked chicken breast, 5 sliced cherry tomatoes, 2 Tbsp. chopped steamed broccoli, 2 Tbsp. sliced red onion, 2 Tbsp. marinara sauce, 2 tsp. dried oregano, 2 tsp. dried basil, 4 slices cooked pepperoni and 2 Tbsp. Parmesan cheese

(8 SUGAR CALORIES, not 403 Calories)

Treat

Up to 2 glasses red wine

(29 SUGAR CALORIES, not 437 Calories)

TOTAL 37 SUGAR CALORIES, not 1739 Calories

Meal Planner: SUNDAY

Breakfast

2 eggs, sunny-side up served over 8 asparagus spears, topped with 1 Tbsp. shaved Parmesan

cheese, served with coffee with half-and-half

(0 SUGAR CALORIES, not 148 Calories)

Snack

¼ cup pumpkin seeds

(0 SUGAR CALORIES, not 71 Calories)

Lunch

Shrimp salad made of 8 cooked baby shrimp mixed with 1 Tbsp. mayo, 2 Tbsp. chopped celery,

1 tsp. lemon juice, 1 tsp. lime juice, and 1 tsp. chopped dill, served on a Romaine lettuce leaf

(0 SUGAR CALORIES, not 151 Calories)

Snack

3 celery sticks spread with cream cheese

(0 SUGAR CALORIES, not 60 Calories)

Dinner

1 chicken breast panfried in 1 Tbsp. olive oil, 1 Tbsp. balsamic vinegar, and 2 tsp. garlic, served

with a side of 6 asparagus spears and 5 cherry tomatoes that have both been drizzled lightly

with balsamic vinegar and cooked in the oven for 10 minutes at 500 degrees, then topped with

8 cubes mozzarella cheese

(12 SUGAR CALORIES, not 311 calories)

Treat

Up to 2 glasses red wine

(29 SUGAR CALORIES, not 437 Calories)

TOTAL 41 SUGAR CALORIES, not 1178 Calories

Shopping List

Produce

60 asparagus spears

25 cherry tomatoes

2 cups arugula

14 celery sticks

lemon juice

lime juice

½ avocado

4 Tbsp. chopped cilantro

3 tsp. chopped dill

4 cups shredded Romaine

5 Romaine leaves

4 Tbsp. chopped green onion

1¼ cup red bell pepper

7 Tbsp. chopped red onion

4 slices onion

1 cup chopped broccoli

3 zucchinis

4 slices eggplant

2 cups mixed greens

garlic

Meat/Fish

2 salmon fillets

5 chicken breasts

12 (1-inch cubes) steak

24 baby shrimp

2 turkey breasts

8 slices pepperoni

Dairy

half-and-half

14 eggs

cream cheese

mozzarella ball

8 Tbsp. Parmesan cheese

¾ cup shredded cheddar cheese

Other

coffee

red wine

vinegar

olive oil

balsamic vinegar

salt

pepper

4 tsp. dried basil

4 tsp. dried oregano

4 Tbsp. marinara sauce

mustard

7 Tbsp. mayonnaise

1 cup pumpkin seeds

¾ cup pecans

The 1 Menu

Breakfast: Omelet made of 2 eggs, ¼ cup shredded Mexican cheese blend, and 2 Tbsp. chunky salsa, served with coffee with half-and-half
(8 SUGAR CALORIES, not 410 Calories)

Snack: 1 handful macadamia nuts
(0 SUGAR CALORIES, not 241 Calories)

Lunch: Season 1 chicken breast with salt and pepper and bake at 400 degrees until cooked through. Whisk together 1 Tbsp. red wine vinegar, 2 tsp. olive oil, and 1 tsp. Dijon mustard, then mix together with chopped cooked chicken breast, 1 cup sliced cucumber, ¼ cup chopped onion, 4 Tbsp. feta cheese crumbles. Serve over 2 cups chopped romaine lettuce.
(0 SUGAR CALORIES, not 309 Calories)

Snack: 1 string cheese stick and 5 almonds
(0 SUGAR CALORIES, not 115 Calories)

Dinner: 1 grilled tilapia fillet, cut into 3 strips, served over 4 Boston lettuce leaves, 1 cup chopped cucumber, ½ cup cilantro sprigs, ¼ cup sliced red pepper, and topped with a mixture of 2 Tbsp. olive oil vinaigrette, 1 tsp. lime juice, and ⅛ tsp. crushed red pepper flakes
(0 SUGAR CALORIES, not 229 Calories)

Treat: Up to 2 glasses red wine
(29 SUGAR CALORIES, not 437 Calories)

TOTAL: 37 SUGAR CALORIES, not 1741 Calories

Options

Breakfast: 1 Skinny Muffin with 2 Tbsp. walnuts (added to the mix) with butter, served with coffee with half-and-half (see page 139 for recipe)

(0 SUGAR CALORIES, not 538 Calories)

Lunch: 1 hamburger patty spread with 1 Tbsp. mustard and topped with 2 slices cheddar cheese, 2 Tbsp. chopped onion, and 3 slices grilled zucchini served on top of 1 cup spinach

(0 SUGAR CALORIES, not 565 Calories)

2 jalapeño peppers sliced in half lengthwise filled with a mixture of 1 Tbsp. creamy goat cheese, 1 Tbsp. cream cheese, 1 Tbsp. grated Parmesan, 1 Tbsp. chopped tomato, and ½ Tbsp. chopped cilantro, each wrapped with 1 slice bacon, secured with a toothpick, and baked for 20 minutes at 375 degrees

(0 SUGAR CALORIES, not 203 Calories)

Dinner: 1 chicken breast seasoned with salt and pepper, sautéed in 1 Tbsp. olive oil, then topped with a mixture of 2 Tbsp. mayo, ¼ cup chopped artichoke hearts, and ⅓ cup grated white cheddar cheese, broiled in the oven for about 3 minutes, or until cheese turns slightly brown, served with a side salad of 1 cup chopped Romaine, 5 halved cherry tomatoes, 1 Tbsp. chopped green onions, with olive oil and vinegar dressing

(0 SUGAR CALORIES, not 711 Calories)

½ large green zucchini cut lengthwise with seeds removed, filled with ¼ pound cooked lean ground turkey (or as much that fits) seasoned with 1 clove chopped garlic, and top with 2 Tbsp. diced tomatoes, 2 Tbsp. chopped onion, and ¼ cup shredded Asiago cheese. Bake in oven at 350 degrees for 45 minutes, or until golden brown. Top with chili flakes, if desired.

(0 SUGAR CALORIES, not 282 Calories)

Snacks: 1 serving deli ham

(0 SUGAR CALORIES, not 46 Calories)

10 almonds

(0 SUGAR CALORIES, not 69 Calories)

Meal Planner: MONDAY

Breakfast

Omelet made of 2 eggs, ¼ cup shredded Mexican cheese blend, and 2 Tbsp. chunky salsa, served with coffee with half-and-half

(8 SUGAR CALORIES, not 410 Calories)

Snack

1 handful macadamia nuts

(0 SUGAR CALORIES, not 241 Calories)

Lunch

Season 1 chicken breast with salt and pepper and bake at 400 degrees until cooked through. Whisk together 1 Tbsp. red wine vinegar, 2 tsp. olive oil, and 1 tsp. Dijon mustard, then mix together with chopped cooked chicken breast, 1 cup sliced cucumber, ¼ cup chopped onion, 4 Tbsp. feta cheese crumbles. Serve all over 2 cups chopped Romaine lettuce.

(0 SUGAR CALORIES, not 309 Calories)

Snack

1 string cheese stick and 5 almonds

(0 SUGAR CALORIES, not 115 Calories)

Dinner

1 grilled tilapia fillet, cut into 3 strips, served over 4 Boston lettuce leafs, 1 cup chopped cucumber, ½ cup cilantro sprigs, ¼ cup sliced red pepper, and topped with a mixture of 2 Tbsp. olive oil vinaigrette, 1 tsp. lime juice, and ⅛ tsp. crushed red pepper flakes

(0 SUGAR CALORIES, not 229 Calories)

Treat

Up to 2 glasses red wine

(29 SUGAR CALORIES, not 437 Calories)

TOTAL 37 SUGAR CALORIES, not 1741 Calories

Meal Planner: TUESDAY

Breakfast

1 Skinny Muffin with 2 Tbsp. walnuts (added to the mix) with butter, served with coffee with half-and-half (see page 139 for recipe)

(0 SUGAR CALORIES, not 538 Calories)

Snack

1 serving deli ham

(0 SUGAR CALORIES, not 46 Calories)

Lunch

1 hamburger spread with 1 Tbsp. mustard and topped with 2 slices cheddar cheese, 2 Tbsp. chopped onion, and 3 slices grilled zucchini served on top of 1 cup spinach

(0 SUGAR CALORIES, not 565 Calories)

Snack

10 almonds

(0 SUGAR CALORIES, not 69 Calories)

Dinner

1 chicken breast seasoned with salt and pepper, sautéed in 1 Tbsp. olive oil, then topped with a mixture of 2 Tbsp. mayo, ¼ cup chopped artichoke hearts, and ⅓ cup grated white cheddar cheese, broiled in the oven for about 3 minutes, or until cheese turns slightly brown, served with a side salad of 1 cup chopped Romaine, 5 halved cherry tomatoes, 1 Tbsp. chopped green onions, with olive oil and vinegar dressing

(0 SUGAR CALORIES, not 711 Calories)

Treat

Up to 2 glasses red wine

(29 SUGAR CALORIES, not 437 Calories)

TOTAL 29 SUGAR CALORIES, not 2366 Calories

Meal Planner: **WEDNESDAY**

Breakfast

Omelet made of 2 eggs, ¼ cup shredded Mexican cheese blend, and 2 Tbsp. chunky salsa,
served with coffee with half-and-half

(8 SUGAR CALORIES, not 410 Calories)

Snack

1 handful macadamia nuts

(0 SUGAR CALORIES, not 241 Calories)

Lunch

2 jalapeño peppers sliced in half lengthwise filled with a mixture of 1 Tbsp. creamy goat cheese,
1 Tbsp. cream cheese, 1 Tbsp. grated Parmesan, 1 Tbsp. chopped tomato, and ½ Tbsp.
chopped cilantro, each wrapped with 1 slice bacon, secured with a toothpick, and baked for
20 minutes at 375 degrees.

(0 SUGAR CALORIES, not 203 Calories)

Snack

1 string cheese stick and 5 almonds

(0 SUGAR CALORIES, not 115 Calories)

Dinner

½ large green zucchini cut lengthwise with seeds removed, filled with ¼ pound cooked lean
ground turkey (or as much that fits) seasoned with 1 clove chopped garlic, and top with 2 Tbsp.
diced tomatoes, 2 Tbsp. chopped onion, and ¼ cup shredded Asiago cheese. Bake in oven at
350 degrees for 45 minutes, or until golden brown. Top with chili flakes, if desired.

(0 SUGAR CALORIES, not 282 Calories)

Treat

Up to 2 glasses red wine

(29 SUGAR CALORIES, not 437 Calories)

TOTAL 37 SUGAR CALORIES, not 1688 Calories

Meal Planner: THURSDAY

Breakfast

1 Skinny Muffin with 2 Tbsp. walnuts (added to the mix) with butter, served with coffee with half-and-half (see page 139 for recipe)

(0 SUGAR CALORIES, not 538 Calories)

Snack

1 serving deli ham

(0 SUGAR CALORIES, not 46 Calories)

Lunch

Season 1 chicken breast with salt and pepper and bake at 400 degrees until cooked through. Whisk together 1 Tbsp. red wine vinegar, 2 tsp. olive oil, and 1 tsp. Dijon mustard, then mix together with chopped cooked chicken breast, 1 cup sliced cucumber, ¼ cup chopped onion, 4 Tbsp. feta cheese crumbles. Serve over 2 cups chopped Romaine lettuce.

(0 SUGAR CALORIES, not 309 Calories)

Snack

10 almonds

(0 SUGAR CALORIES, not 69 Calories)

Dinner

1 grilled tilapia fillet, cut into 3 strips, served over 4 Boston lettuce leafs, 1 cup chopped cucumber, ½ cup cilantro sprigs, ¼ cup sliced red pepper, and topped with a mixture of 2 Tbsp. olive oil vinaigrette, 1 tsp. lime juice, and ⅛ tsp. crushed red pepper flakes

(0 SUGAR CALORIES, not 229 Calories)

Treat

Up to 2 glasses red wine

(29 SUGAR CALORIES, not 437 Calories)

TOTAL 29 SUGAR CALORIES, not 1628 Calories

Meal Planner: FRIDAY

Breakfast

Omelet made of 2 eggs, ¼ cup shredded Mexican cheese blend, and 2 Tbsp. chunky salsa, served with coffee with half-and-half

(8 SUGAR CALORIES, not 410 Calories)

Snack

1 handful macadamia nuts

(0 SUGAR CALORIES, not 241 Calories)

Lunch

1 hamburger spread with 1 Tbsp. mustard and topped with 2 slices cheddar cheese, 2 Tbsp. chopped onion, and 3 slices grilled zucchini served on top of 1 cup spinach

(0 SUGAR CALORIES, not 565 Calories)

Snack

1 string cheese stick and 5 almonds

(0 SUGAR CALORIES, not 115 Calories)

Dinner

1 chicken breast seasoned with salt and pepper, sautéed in 1 Tbsp. olive oil, then topped with a mixture of 2 Tbsp. mayo, ¼ cup chopped artichoke hearts, and ⅓ cup grated white cheddar cheese, broiled in the oven for about 3 minutes, or until cheese turns slightly brown, served with a side salad of 1 cup chopped Romaine, 5 halved cherry tomatoes, 1 Tbsp. chopped green onions, with olive oil and vinegar dressing

(0 SUGAR CALORIES, not 711 Calories)

Treat

Up to 2 glasses red wine

(29 SUGAR CALORIES, not 437 Calories)

TOTAL 37 SUGAR CALORIES, not 2479 Calories

Meal Planner: **SATURDAY**

Breakfast

1 Skinny Muffin with 2 Tbsp. walnuts (added to the mix) with butter, served with coffee with half-and-half (see page 139 for recipe)

(0 SUGAR CALORIES, not 538 Calories)

Snack

1 serving deli ham

(0 SUGAR CALORIES, not 46 Calories)

Lunch

2 jalapeño peppers sliced in half lengthwise filled with a mixture of 1 Tbsp. creamy goat cheese, 1 Tbsp. cream cheese, 1 Tbsp. grated Parmesan, 1 Tbsp. chopped tomato, and ½ Tbsp. chopped cilantro, each wrapped with 1 slice bacon, secured with a toothpick, and baked for 20 minutes at 375 degrees

(0 SUGAR CALORIES, not 203 Calories)

Snack

10 almonds

(0 SUGAR CALORIES, not 69 Calories)

Dinner

½ large green zucchini cut lengthwise with seeds removed, filled with ¼ pound cooked lean ground turkey (or as much that fits) seasoned with 1 clove chopped garlic, and top with 2 Tbsp. diced tomatoes, 2 Tbsp. chopped onion, and ¼ cup shredded Asiago cheese. Bake in oven at 350 degrees for 45 minutes, or until golden brown. Top with chili flakes, if desired.

(0 SUGAR CALORIES, not 282 Calories)

Treat

Up to 2 glasses red wine

(29 SUGAR CALORIES, not 437 Calories)

TOTAL 29 SUGAR CALORIES, not 1575 Calories

Meal Planner: **SUNDAY**

Breakfast

Omelet made of 2 eggs, ¼ cup shredded Mexican cheese blend, and 2 Tbsp. chunky salsa, served with coffee with half-and-half

(8 SUGAR CALORIES, not 410 Calories)

Snack

1 handful macadamia nuts

(0 SUGAR CALORIES, not 241 Calories)

Lunch

Season 1 chicken breast with salt and pepper and bake at 400 degrees until cooked through. Whisk together 1 Tbsp. red wine vinegar, 2 tsp. olive oil, and 1 tsp. Dijon mustard, then mix together with chopped cooked chicken breast, 1 cup sliced cucumber, ¼ cup chopped onion, 4 Tbsp. feta cheese crumbles. Serve over 2 cups chopped Romaine lettuce.

(0 SUGAR CALORIES, not 309 Calories)

Snack

1 string cheese stick and 5 almonds

(0 SUGAR CALORIES, not 115 Calories)

Dinner

1 grilled tilapia fillet, cut into 3 strips, served over 4 Boston lettuce leafs, 1 cup chopped cucumber, ½ cup cilantro sprigs, ¼ cup sliced red pepper, and topped with a mixture of 2 Tbsp. olive oil vinaigrette, 1 tsp. lime juice, and ⅛ tsp. crushed red pepper flakes

(0 SUGAR CALORIES, not 229 Calories)

Treat

Up to 2 glasses red wine

(29 SUGAR CALORIES, not 437 Calories)

TOTAL 37 SUGAR CALORIES, not 1741 Calories

Shopping List

Produce

4 jalapeño peppers	2 large zucchinis	6 Tbsp. diced tomatoes
6 cups cucumber	½ cup artichoke hearts	10 cherry tomatoes
cilantro	8 cups Romaine lettuce	2 onions
3 tsp. lime juice	2 cups spinach	2 Tbsp. green onion
2 cloves garlic	12 Boston lettuce leaves	¾ cup sliced red bell pepper

Meat/Fish

3 tilapia fillets	2 hamburger patties	3 servings deli ham
5 chicken breasts	½ lb. lean ground turkey	4 strips bacon

Dairy

half-and-half	12 Tbsp. feta cheese crumbles	2 Tbsp. cream cheese
butter		2 Tbsp. Parmesan cheese
12 eggs	4 slices cheddar cheese	½ cup Asiago cheese
4 string cheese sticks	2 Tbsp. creamy goat cheese	⅔ cup white cheddar cheese
1 cup Mexican cheese blend		

Other

coffee	8 tsp. cinnamon powder	3 tsp. Dijon mustard
red wine		2 Tbsp. mustard
vinegar	coconut oil	chili flakes
olive oil	baking powder	crushed red pepper flakes
red wine vinegar	8 Tbsp. chunky salsa	
salt	6 Tbsp. walnuts	4 Tbsp. mayonnaise
pepper	macadamia nuts (about 4 handfuls)	
4 packets Stevia/Truvia		
1 cup ground flax	50 almonds	

The 1 Menu

Breakfast: 2 fried eggs served with 2 breakfast sausage links and coffee with half-and-half
(0 SUGAR CALORIES, not 335 Calories)

Snack: ¼ cup sunflower seeds
(0 SUGAR CALORIES, not 186 Calories)

Lunch: 1 turkey burger spread with 1 Tbsp. mustard, topped with 1 slice melted American cheese, 1 slice tomato, 2 rings of grilled onions, 5 grilled mushroom slices, all served on 2 Bibb lettuce leaves
(0 SUGAR CALORIES, not 266 calories)

Snack: 1 hard-boiled egg
(0 SUGAR CALORIES, not 80 Calories)

Dinner: 1 chicken breast, cut into strips, sautéed in a pan with 1 Tbsp. olive oil, 1 Tbsp. chopped garlic, 1 cup chopped broccoli, mixed with ¼ cup alfredo sauce and topped with 2 Tbsp. Parmesan cheese
(12 SUGAR CALORIES, not 435 Calories)

Treat: Up to 2 glasses red wine
(29 SUGAR CALORIES, not 437 Calories)

TOTAL: 41 SUGAR CALORIES, not 1739 Calories

Options

Breakfast: 1 cup cottage cheese mixed with ¼ cup chopped walnuts, served with coffee with half-and-half
(0 SUGAR CALORIES, not 395 Calories)

Lunch: 2 1-inch thick slices of eggplant, brushed with olive oil and roasted at 375 degrees for about 18–20 minutes, then each topped with 2 Tbsp. marinara sauce, 1 Tbsp. chopped basil, and ¼ cup grated mozzarella cheese and broiled until cheese is melted
(8 SUGAR CALORIES, not 107 Calories)

1 cup shredded Romaine lettuce, topped with ¼ cup shredded deli turkey, 1 Tbsp. Parmesan cheese, and 2 Tbsp. Caesar dressing
(4 SUGAR CALORIES, not 277 Calories)

Dinner: 2 steak kebabs each made from 3 1-inch pieces grilled steak, 3 slices grilled red bell pepper, 3 slices grilled zucchini, and 2 grilled mushrooms
(0 SUGAR CALORIES, not 211 Calories)

1 grilled chicken breast, topped with 1 slice fresh mozzarella, 2 basil leaves, and 1 slice tomato, drizzled in 2 Tbsp. balsamic vinegar
(16 SUGAR CALORIES, not 209 Calories)

Snacks: 10 almonds and 1 string cheese stick
(0 SUGAR CALORIES, not 149 Calories)

5 cucumber slices topped with cream cheese
(0 SUGAR CALORIES, not 109 Calories)

Meal Planner: MONDAY

Breakfast

2 fried eggs served with 2 breakfast sausage links and coffee with half-and-half

(0 SUGAR CALORIES, not 335 Calories)

Snack

¼ cup sunflower seeds

(0 SUGAR CALORIES, not 186 Calories)

Lunch

1 turkey burger spread with 1 Tbsp. mustard, topped with 1 slice melted American cheese,

1 slice tomato, 2 rings of grilled onions, 5 grilled mushroom slices, all served on 2 Bibb lettuce

leaves

(0 SUGAR CALORIES, not 266 Calories)

Snack

1 hard-boiled egg

(0 SUGAR CALORIES, not 80 Calories)

Dinner

1 chicken breast, cut into strips, sautéed in a pan with 1 Tbsp. olive oil, 1 Tbsp. chopped garlic,

1 cup chopped broccoli, mixed with ¼ cup alfredo sauce and topped with 2 Tbsp. Parmesan

cheese

(12 SUGAR CALORIES, not 435 Calories)

Treat

Up to 2 glasses red wine

(29 SUGAR CALORIES, not 437 Calories)

TOTAL 41 SUGAR CALORIES, not 1739 Calories

Meal Planner: **TUESDAY**

Breakfast

1 cup cottage cheese mixed with ¼ cup chopped walnuts, served with coffee with half-and-half

(0 SUGAR CALORIES, not 395 Calories)

Snack

10 almonds and 1 string cheese stick

(0 SUGAR CALORIES, not 149 Calories)

Lunch

2 1-inch thick slices of eggplant, brushed with olive oil and roasted at 375 degrees for about 18–20 minutes, then each topped with 2 Tbsp. marinara sauce, 1 Tbsp. chopped basil, and ¼ cup grated mozzarella cheese and broiled until cheese is melted

(8 SUGAR CALORIES, not 107 Calories)

Snack

5 cucumber slices topped with cream cheese

(0 SUGAR CALORIES, not 109 Calories)

Dinner

2 steak kebabs each made from 3 1-inch pieces grilled steak, 3 slices grilled red bell pepper, 3 slices grilled zucchini, and 2 grilled mushrooms

(0 SUGAR CALORIES, not 211 Calories)

Treat

Up to 2 glasses red wine

(29 SUGAR CALORIES, not 437 Calories)

TOTAL 37 SUGAR CALORIES, not 1408 Calories

Meal Planner: WEDNESDAY

Breakfast

2 fried eggs served with 2 breakfast sausage links and coffee with half-and-half

(0 SUGAR CALORIES, not 335 Calories)

Snack

¼ cup sunflower seeds

(0 SUGAR CALORIES, not 186 Calories)

Lunch

1 cup shredded Romaine lettuce, topped with ¼ cup shredded deli turkey, 1 Tbsp. Parmesan cheese, and 2 Tbsp. Caesar dressing

(4 SUGAR CALORIES, not 277 Calories)

Snack

1 hard-boiled egg

(0 SUGAR CALORIES, not 80 Calories)

Dinner

1 grilled chicken breast, topped with 1 slice fresh mozzarella, 2 basil leaves, and 1 slice tomato, drizzled in 2 Tbsp. balsamic vinegar

(16 SUGAR CALORIES, not 209 Calories)

Treat

Up to 2 glasses red wine

(29 SUGAR CALORIES, not 437 Calories)

TOTAL 49 SUGAR CALORIES, not 1524 Calories

Meal Planner: **THURSDAY**

Breakfast

1 cup cottage cheese mixed with ¼ cup chopped walnuts, served with coffee with half-and-half

(0 SUGAR CALORIES, not 395 Calories)

Snack

10 almonds and 1 string cheese stick

(0 SUGAR CALORIES, not 149 Calories)

Lunch

1 turkey burger spread with 1 Tbsp. mustard, topped with 1 slice melted American cheese,

1 slice tomato, 2 rings of grilled onions, 5 grilled mushroom slices, all served on 2 Bibb lettuce

leaves

(0 SUGAR CALORIES, not 266 Calories)

Snack

5 cucumber slices topped with cream cheese

(0 SUGAR CALORIES, not 109 Calories)

Dinner

1 chicken breast, cut into strips, sautéed in a pan with 1 Tbsp. olive oil, 1 Tbsp. chopped garlic,

1 cup chopped broccoli, mixed with ¼ cup alfredo sauce and topped with 2 Tbsp. Parmesan

cheese

(12 SUGAR CALORIES, not 435 Calories)

Treat

Up to 2 glasses red wine

(29 SUGAR CALORIES, not 437 Calories)

TOTAL 41 SUGAR CALORIES, not 1791 Calories

Meal Planner: FRIDAY

Breakfast

2 fried eggs served with 2 breakfast sausage links and coffee with half-and-half

(0 SUGAR CALORIES, not 335 Calories)

Snack

¼ cup sunflower seeds

(0 SUGAR CALORIES, not 186 Calories)

Lunch

2 1-inch thick slices of eggplant, brushed with olive oil and roasted at 375 degrees for about 18–20 minutes, then each topped with 2 Tbsp. marinara sauce, 1 Tbsp. chopped basil, and ¼ cup grated mozzarella cheese and broiled until cheese is melted

(8 SUGAR CALORIES, not 107 Calories)

Snack

1 hard-boiled egg

(0 SUGAR CALORIES, not 80 Calories)

Dinner

2 steak kebabs each made from 3 1-inch pieces grilled steak, 3 slices grilled red bell pepper, 3 slices grilled zucchini, and 2 grilled mushrooms

(0 SUGAR CALORIES, not 211 Calories)

Treat

Up to 2 glasses red wine

(29 SUGAR CALORIES, not 437 Calories)

TOTAL 37 SUGAR CALORIES, not 1356 Calories

Meal Planner: **SATURDAY**

Breakfast

1 cup cottage cheese mixed with ¼ cup chopped walnuts, served with coffee with half-and-half

(0 SUGAR CALORIES, not 395 Calories)

Snack

10 almonds and 1 string cheese stick

(0 SUGAR CALORIES, not 149 Calories)

Lunch

1 cup shredded Romaine lettuce, topped with ¼ cup shredded deli turkey, 1 Tbsp. Parmesan cheese, and 2 Tbsp. Caesar dressing

(4 SUGAR CALORIES, not 277 Calories)

Snack

5 cucumber slices topped with cream cheese

(0 SUGAR CALORIES, not 109 Calories)

Dinner

1 grilled chicken breast, topped with 1 slice fresh mozzarella, 2 basil leaves, and 1 slice tomato, drizzled in 2 Tbsp. balsamic vinegar

(16 SUGAR CALORIES, not 209 Calories)

Treat

Up to 2 glasses red wine

(29 SUGAR CALORIES, not 437 Calories)

TOTAL 49 SUGAR CALORIES, not 1576 Calories

Meal Planner: SUNDAY

Breakfast

2 fried eggs served with 2 breakfast sausage links and coffee with half-and-half

(0 SUGAR CALORIES, not 335 Calories)

Snack

¼ cup sunflower seeds

(0 SUGAR CALORIES, not 186 Calories)

Lunch

1 turkey burger spread with 1 Tbsp. mustard, topped with 1 slice melted American cheese,
1 slice tomato, 2 rings of grilled onions, 5 grilled mushroom slices, all served on 2 Bibb lettuce
leaves

(0 SUGAR CALORIES, not 266 Calories)

Snack

1 hard-boiled egg

(0 SUGAR CALORIES, not 80 Calories)

Dinner

1 chicken breast, cut into strips, sautéed in a pan with 1 Tbsp. olive oil, 1 Tbsp. chopped garlic,
1 cup chopped broccoli, mixed with ¼ cup alfredo sauce and topped with 2 Tbsp. Parmesan
cheese

(12 SUGAR CALORIES, not 435 Calories)

Treat

Up to 2 glasses red wine

(29 SUGAR CALORIES, not 437 Calories)

TOTAL 41 SUGAR CALORIES, not 1739 Calories

Shopping List

Produce

15 cucumber slices	6 Bibb/butter lettuce	3 Tbsp. garlic
5 slices tomato	leaves	3 cups broccoli
6 rings/slices onion	2 cups shredded	
19 mushroom slices	Romaine lettuce	

Meat/Fish

8 breakfast sausage links	¼ cup shredded deli	4 (1-inch thick) slices
5 chicken breasts	turkey	eggplant
3 turkey burger patties	fresh basil	6 slices red bell pepper
12 (1-inch-thick) steak		6 slices zucchini
cubes		

Dairy

half-and-half	3 string cheese sticks	½ cup grated mozzarella
12 eggs	cream cheese	3 slices American cheese
3 cups cottage cheese	2 slices fresh mozzarella	8 Tbsp. Parmesan cheese

Other

coffee	salt	30 almonds
red wine	pepper	3 Tbsp. mustard
vinegar	¾ cup chopped	4 Tbsp. marinara
olive oil	walnuts	sauce
balsamic vinegar	1 cup sunflower seeds	¾ cup alfredo sauce

Skinny Muffin Recipe

¼ cup ground flax

1 tsp. baking powder

2 tsp. cinnamon powder

1 tsp. coconut oil

1 egg

1 packet Stevia/Truvia

* Makes 1 Skinny Muffin

Mix all ingredients together in a coffee mug. Microwave for 50 seconds.

THE **100** | Conclusion

Congratulations. You've completed the first four weeks of your new way of life. Now it's time to make a choice. You can either continue on by simply repeating the menus outlined in this chapter, or you can follow the suggestions you'll find in the next chapter. The choice is yours.

JORGE: Is sugar a type of opiate?

GARY: [Sugars and refined carbohydrates] affect that part of the brain that other drugs of abuse do. That is pretty clear. The cravings are powerful. The question is you don't really want to play games with this. You don't want to figure out loopholes– when you want to quit smoking you don't ask your doctor, "Well, can I smoke three of those Indian cigarettes a day?" If you are trying to quit drinking you don't say, "Okay, I am going to give up the vodka and the tequila, but I am going to allow myself half a bottle of wine twice a week." You know you are pretty much doomed to fail. And so I take a kind of hard line view on it. This is serious health problems. As serious as any health problem you can have. You know, take a hard line approach to it. Can you eat fruit? Maybe.

JORGE: If there were two fruits, three fruits you could recommend what would they be? How about an avocado?

GARY: Yes. Avocados are probably fine.

JORGE: They have the fats for our skin and appetite.

GARY: The thing to remember is that carbohydrates stimulate hunger. There is a difference. The fats in foods don't do this. When you stimulate insulin you stimulate hunger. So, avocados, they are high in fat, and relatively low carbohydrate. After that you are getting into difficult games [with other fruits].

JORGE: Berries, you said some berries?

GARY: Well, blueberries, you know, some low-carb diet doctors like—again, you are pushing me to treat it like, Indian cigarettes. How about just a joint every now and then? What can I smoke? You know, if you want to lose weight, take it seriously. Then you can see. If you get rid of most of these, all of the sugars and most of the carbs, most of the refined carbs, you are eating a lot of green, leafy vegetables, a lot of things that are good for you.

JORGE: So the fruits we should be eating aren't fruits, they are vegetables?

GARY: Yea, yea.

JORGE: It's a swap, if you will.

GARY: The starches are swapped for vegetables as well. Instead of having broccoli, potatoes and fish you have broccoli, broccoli and fish. Instead of spinach, rice and meat you have spinach, spinach, and meat, or spinach, a salad, and meat. You can always, especially if you go into restaurants, you can say hold the potatoes. Give me an extra serving of vegetables.

" I DID IT ! "

ALICIA

VITAL STATS

AGE: 41   **HEIGHT:** 5' 8"   **WEIGHT LOST:** 27 pounds

MY BEST STRATEGY: Be patient. I learned that just because my weight loss might slow one week, didn't mean I was doing anything wrong. I kept close to the menus, and accepted that sometimes my body's wisdom needed to slow down progress—but the weight does come off, and by limiting my Sugar Calories, it stays off!

PART THREE

What's Next

Beyond the fact that diets are flawed from the get-go, another reason we tend to stray from our new patterns is we have not properly developed new and sustainable routines in life. If one of your new goals is to become a dancer, you may start taking a dance class, but, in order for you to be a skilled and elegant dancer you need to take the steps from the ballroom into your daily routine, daydream about it, stop and notice when others are doing it, and dance constantly. Basically to be a great dancer, dancing needs to be a part of you. The secret is immersion.

For the next couple of chapters I am going to get you immersed in the world of health by taking the four week plan you completed and making it a lifestyle. I will give you the instruction to really make this program live outside of the simple idea written down in this book. I know that you will be able to take this information and have it become automatic, with no-think eating and all the bonuses that come from being healthy. Chapter 6 has all the tools needed to get motivated and stay there, giving you confidence that soars with my practical tips and application. Get ready to conquer any obstacle thrown in your new path to health.

5

Week Five and Beyond

The greatest revolution of our generation is
the discovery that human beings, by changing the inner attitudes of their minds, can
change the outer aspects of their lives.

—WILLIAM JAMES

If you have finished the first four weeks of The 100™ menus, congratulations to you! Please share your success at Facebook.com/JorgeCruiseFan and help cheer more on. However, my guess is that you peaked ahead to this chapter before you finished with the menus, and that's great. People who think ahead how they will continue to succeed are more likely to do so. Here's where you can start to think about the steps you'll take. When you do come to your fifth week you get to make a choice.

THE 100 | Option 1: Let ME Be Your Coach

If you are busy or looking for more variety without having to develop and create them, you can get more menus and recipes at my website, JorgeCruise.com, and have me do all the work for you with my online program. I'll provide you with new menus each week, so you never have repetitive meals, and you'll always have access to easy to make, delicious foods that follow The 100™. Studies have shown that when people are coached they are able to lose three times more weight. That is the main reason I have developed an online resource where I can be your coach and give you new meals and meal planners that will take the stress out of weight control. If you are serious about making the change I invite you to see what my online program has to offer at JorgeCruise.com. If this is the option that fits your lifestyle I look forward to working with you.

THE 100 | Option 2: Let the BOOK Coach You

You can also simply return to the first four weeks in chapter 4 and follow the menus again. For some there is great power in simplicity. If you enjoy a very structured routine you may find that knowing exactly what to eat each week from the guidelines in this book are a perfect fit for your lifestyle. However, if you are feeling adventurous check out . . .

You can read on and learn how to take your new knowledge to the next level and start making your own menus from the food lists located in the bonus chapters I have included. To create your own meals and menus, see the chart on the following page for easy tracking of your foods. Remember to just mark down your Sugar Calories and to keep them under 100 per day. For the fastest weight loss, choose the healthiest Sugar Calories and save those with the highest levels of sugars and refined flours for special treat days. In addition, make sure you include plenty of Vegetable Freebies from the Freebie lists starting on page 170. The high fiber in the foods will help you feel full and satisfied, and will help you lose weight faster. Finally, the initial building blocks of any meal should be proteins and fats because these are the two nutrients that satisfy your hunger best and take the longest to digest, so you feel full for longer amounts of time. Plus, proteins and fats don't spike insulin levels, so you'll never feel like you're starving, you won't have cravings for those fattening carbohydrates, and your body will naturally use more of your stored fat as fuel.

Let's look at a sample meal to see how you'd track your Sugar Calories and Freebies if you are aiming to stay at 100 Sugar Calories per day:

Doing It Yourself

Meal: Breakfast	Freebies	Sugar Calories
2 scrambled eggs	yes	0
2 sausage patties	yes	0
Meal: Snack	**Freebies**	**Sugar Calories**
1 string cheese	yes	0
Meal: Lunch	**Freebies**	**Sugar Calories**
1 slice, bread, Food For Life Sprouted Grain Ezekiel 4:9 Bread	no	60
1 slice Swiss cheese, 1 oz.	yes	0
Ground turkey patty, 3 oz. cooked, 85% lean	yes	0
Lettuce, tomato	yes	0
Mayonnaise, 1 Tbsp.	yes	0
Meal: Snack	**Freebies**	**Sugar Calories**
11 almonds, dry roasted	yes	0
¼ cup blueberries	yes	22
Meal: Dinner	**Freebies**	**Sugar Calories**
Ricotta cheese, part skim ¼ cup	yes	0
Prosciutto, 4 slices, 2 oz. diced	yes	0
Parmesan cheese, 1 Tbsp.	yes	0
Chopped tomato and spinach, 1 cup	yes	0
Meal: Dessert	**Freebies**	**Sugar Calories**
1 Joseph's Sugar-Free Crispy Bite Size Cookie	no	13
Totals for day		**95**

As you can see, all you have to do is look up the carb grams in the food and multiply it by 4 to get your Sugar Calories—or look for your food on my food lists in chapter 8.

Now it's your turn! On the next page, there is a chart you can use and make copies of for planning out your own meals and menus. While you don't

Meal: Breakfast	Freebies	Sugar Calories (Carb grams X 4, rounded, or use food lists)
Meal: Snack	Freebies	Sugar Calories
Meal: Lunch	Freebies	Sugar Calories
Meal: Snack	Freebies	Sugar Calories
Meal: Dinner	Freebies	Sugar Calories
Meal: Dessert	Freebies	Sugar Calories
Totals for day		

*Note: For tracking your Sugar Calories—if you are eating a food that is not on the provided food lists look at the label and determine the amount of Sugar Calories by multiplying the carb grams on the label by 4.

need to track anything other than your Sugar Calories, research does show that keeping a food diary can help you be more aware of the food choices you are making, helping you to be more conscious about what you are putting in your mouth. So keep a loose list of what your meals and snacks are, and be sure to tally your Sugar Calories and keep to the 100 calorie limit.

THE 100 | Conclusion

Well done. You now have all the tools for creating a lifetime of eating that will help you lose weight and maintain your new slim figure. Not only do you have a structured four week plan but you also have plenty of variety to choose from the tools to create your own menus by using the food lists in chapter 8.

In the next chapter, I'll introduce strategies for staying motivated, and be sure to check out the appendices in the back of the book for information and resources to keep you going.

MARY ANNE

VITAL STATS

AGE: 43   **HEIGHT:** 5' 5"   **WEIGHT LOST:** 42 pounds

MY BEST STRATEGY: Being creative with my meals, and enjoying treats. I love to try out new recipes and spices to mix things up for my taste buds. Not getting caught up in the same three meals every day helps me stay motivated to stick to my goals. There's so much you can make or adapt to this way of eating. One of my favorite things to make is an easy coconut Thai soup with chicken. I mix one can of coconut milk, 2 tablespoons of red curry paste (in the Asian section of your supermarket) with 3 cups of chicken broth—whisk this together on the stove with some salt and pepper and you have a great base for a quick soup. Just add some chopped cooked chicken (a rotisserie chicken from the grocery store is a fast fix), some sliced snow peas, chopped tomatoes, and fresh chopped cilantro and a squeeze of lemon for garnish and flavor, and you're good to go. My favorite treat is to whip up some heavy whipping cream with a bit of stevia and cinnamon and top some sliced strawberries with it. Delicious.

I used to have to take more and more thyroid medicine for a condition I have, but my doctor said I could decrease it after eating this way. It's so great to need less, rather than more of a drug. I know I can easily eat this way for the rest of my life—and so can my family.

"I DID IT!"

ELIZABETH

VITAL STATS

AGE: 50   **HEIGHT:** 5' 9"   **WEIGHT LOST:** 70 pounds

MY BEST STRATEGY: Be prepared! I never leave home without a snack, and I have plenty of nosh-worthy foods in my fridge. That way I always have a good choice within arm's reach. String cheese, walnuts, almonds, cucumber slices are a girl's best friend. Before I found Jorge I felt like I was ready to lose weight, but I just didn't know how. Life since I've changed my eating habits has been amazing. I gave up sugar, and since then I feel empowered and confident. Jorge opened my eyes to all the ways traditional diets can sabotage you even when you are trying your very best to follow all the rules. This philosophy of eating is so simple. Today I'm confident in how I look and feel, and I now know that I can accomplish any of my dreams.

Motivational Tools

It is our attitude at the beginning of a difficult
task which, more than anything else, will
affect its successful outcome.

—WILLIAM JAMES

To stay motivated about any new diet and food plan takes more than just
following a menu. Being prepared with strategies and tips for keeping
motivation strong can keep you on track through even the most difficult times.
Read on for my favorite ways of troubleshooting obstacles and best tips for staying inspired to stick to your goals. You'll also find the most common answers to
frequently asked questions below.

1. Use a mantra: Use a mantra to get you through moments of difficulty. A mantra is a phrase that is repeated either out loud or silently to yourself to verbalize and visualize what you want.

"I can do this. I am strong."

"I eat to live, I don't live to eat."

"I am healthy and fit."

"One day at a time."

"This too shall pass."

2. Create a power photo collage. Make a collage of images and pictures that inspire you. The collages help you to visually commit to losing weight.

3. Clean out the clutter. Take inventory of your cupboards, refrigerator, or even your secret stash of snacks. Then designate one master area that is not easy for you to reach for the foods that are your biggest weakness. Sometimes it is above the microwave or cupboard above the fridge because it is nice and out of the way. If you need to, inform those in your house where you have moved these foods, so they are not constantly asking where the chips have gone.

4. Review your motivation daily. People doing the best have a specific motivation for losing weight. It might be an upcoming occasion, or the desire to be fit enough to play with your grandchildren. Remind yourself daily about this reason, whatever it is.

5. Find three supportive teammates. If you want to lose weight, enlist support. It's a lonely job, losing weight. People often find comfort in food. We should really be finding comfort in friends and family. You need support. Have three people that you can touch base with every day in order to maintain a regimen of support. By establishing a support network of people to help you on your journey you'll guarantee your success. This team can include family members, co-workers, and good friends—anyone you feel comfortable talking with openly and honestly. Choose teammates who are nonjudgmental, willing to listen, and be supportive. Designate one person as your email buddy, one as a phone buddy, and one person as your accountability buddy. This last person will help you stay true to your goals by talking to you every day, even if it is just for a quick check in. It's important to make sure that your accountability buddy is someone you admire and strive to be like.

6. Sign a contract: Making a commitment in writing is an easy way to ramp up your motivation. Sign the one on the following page and post it where you can see it.

The 100™ Success Contract

I, _____, commit to following The 100™ menus and principles for the next four weeks, because I am worth it. I am committed to loving myself and my body.

My motivation is

_____

_____

My designated buddies are:

Email Buddy _____

Phone Buddy _____

Accountability Buddy _____

Signature _____

I love quotes. I find that they can sum up a thought or a wisdom that could take chapters to write in just a few words. In addition to the quotes found at the beginning of each of the chapters in this book, here are some of my other favorite quotes that can be used when life gets tough. **I suggest picking one of these to use as a daily motivator or mantra. Write it on a sticky note and post it where you can see it.**

Progress is impossible without change and those who cannot change their minds cannot change anything.

—GEORGE BERNARD SHAW

If you change the way you look at things, the things you look at change.

—WAYNE DYER

Little by little does the trick.

—AESOP

We must be the change we wish to see in the world.

—MAHATMA GANDHI

One may walk over the highest mountain one step at a time.

—JOHN WANAMAKER

Whether you think you can or can't, you're right.

—HENRY FORD

Stumbling is not falling.

—PORTUGUESE PROVERB

You are braver than you believe, stronger than you seem, and smarter than you think.

—CHRISTOPHER ROBIN

It's in your moments of decision that your destiny is shaped.

—ANTHONY ROBBINS

Don't wait until everything is just right. It will never be perfect. There will always be challenges, obstacles and less than perfect conditions. So what. Get started now. With each step you take, you will grow stronger and stronger, more and more skilled, more and more self-confident and more and more successful.

—MARK VICTOR HANSEN

It's not the mistakes in life that are important; it's what we learn from them.

—DONNA GUTHRIE

Two roads diverged in a wood, and I . . . I took the one less traveled by, and that has made all the difference.

—ROBERT FROST

What else can I do to stay motivated?

Along with the tools outlined in this book, I encourage you to check out my website, www.JorgeCruise.com, for fantastic tips and strategies for healthy eating that will help you lose and keep the weight off for good. At my website, you can join my free email club and get more advice for free as well as follow me on my social sites to get more tips and application. From time to time I do offer more ways to be coached by me, whether it is by more recipes, meal planners, or live sessions to get you on track. Be sure to check out my site to see which program of mine is right for you.

"I DID IT!"

MELANIE

VITALS

AGE: 46   **HEIGHT:** 5' 7"   **WEIGHT LOST:** 20 pounds

BEST STRATEGY: Bake ahead of time. I love to cook up a bunch of chicken breasts at one time. You can either throw them in a baking pan and cook them in the oven, or put them in a big pan and cover them with water (add salt, pepper, a couple bay leaves, and a chopped onion), and bring to a boil, then turn down the heat and simmer for about 90 minutes. Strain—you have plenty of chicken and broth as a bonus for upcoming meals. I'll use these over several days sliced up over a salad for lunches, stir fried with broccoli for dinners, or in a quesadilla. Yum.

I was really skeptical when I started this plan because I was still able to make room for ice cream and chocolate, but after one week I was blown away by losing seven pounds. I used to feel so bloated and fatigued, now I am trim and full of energy. I know I feel so much better because I was able to set aside my horrible sugar habit. I had no idea I was eating upward of 200 grams of sugar a day.

PART FOUR

Bonus Material

> Yesterday's the past, tomorrow's the future, but today is a gift. That's why it's called the present.
> —BIL KEANE

Who doesn't like a bonus now and again? If you are really ready to make a big shift in your life the next bonus chapters are perfect for you. In the next three chapters you will find some valuable tools that help you fit into a new lifestyle and be truly liberated. First up is The 100™ Plus plan for days when you may need a little more of the smart Sugar Calories, I'll teach you how to add a little more and still have success each week. There is also a more structured plan if you need to take the weekends off. Then the reveal of The 100™ Food List, a comprehensive list of Freebies you can enjoy whenever you are venturing away from the meal planners and you are making your meals your own. You will also see the Sugar Calories in other foods, some are shocking but at the same time you will see how easy it is to make this a lifestyle.

What diet book is complete without a full and drawn-out workout routine? This book is! No workout routine required, and as you will learn you are doing yourself a favor by not being tied to the gym and working out for several hours a day. But fear not, don't think I am being unreasonable here, I actually give you the right guidelines on how to be active that are surprisingly fun and easy. What are you waiting for? Go get those bonuses!

7

When to Add More Sugar Calories

Do the best you can, and don't take life too
serious.

—WILL ROGERS

Sometimes life is messy and overwhelming, sometimes your schedule is
overflowing with parties, dining out, or weekend barbecues. At these
times, you may feel like The 100™ limit on your Sugar Calories just isn't going
to work for you.

Some of my clients, especially women over 40, are concerned about severe
carbohydrate cravings. Some of this may be related to hormone fluctuations
and can be remedied by an increase in carbohydrates. But you don't have to
just throw in the towel. You can still lose weight, albeit at a more modified
pace, with a few more Sugar Calories. That's where the two following strategies come into play. The first is The 100™ Plus, which accommodates up to
300 Sugar Calories a day, while the second is a weekend plan that has you follow The 100™ for the week, and then allows you more Sugar Calories on the
weekends. Both of these options still limit your Sugar Calories so you can lose
weight, but allow you to have more smart sugars at the same time.

The 100™ offers you the fastest, most satisfying weight loss plan ever, and my hope is that you'll feel comfortable following this strategy until you reach your weight loss goal. That said, there may be times when you feel you'd like to add a few more smart sugars into your diet, while still moving toward your weight loss goals. That's fine. The reality is that when you up your smart sugar level you will get more Sugar Calories, but I've found that as long as you keep these under 300 Sugar Calories a day, you will still see weight loss, just at a slightly slower rate of 1 to 2 pounds per week, which is still great.

To follow the 100™ Plus, you can use the food planner below, and the food lists in the next chapter. You'll just be tracking up to 300 Sugar Calories per day. You don't need to eat all 300—this should be your maximum. I call them smart sugars because you should choose from the healthiest Sugar Calories, which contain the highest levels of fiber, vitamins, minerals, and antioxidants. Here is my recommendation towards which Sugar Calories you should choose:

1. Beans and legumes

2. Starchy vegetables

3. Whole grains

4. Fruits

5. Refined carbs (white bread, buns, rolls)

6. Condiments

7. Treats and desserts

The 100 Plus Menu Tracker

Meal: Breakfast	Freebies	Sugar Calories (Carb grams X 4, rounded, or use food lists)
Meal: Snack	**Freebies**	**Sugar Calories**
Meal: Lunch	**Freebies**	**Sugar Calories**
Meal: Snack	**Freebies**	**Sugar Calories**
Meal: Dinner	**Freebies**	**Sugar Calories**
Totals for day		

The Weekend Planner

Your other option is to follow The 100™ to limit your Sugar Calories from Monday through Friday, and then follow The 100™ Plus, or the sample menu below.

Weekend Menu

Breakfast: 1 small baguette, toasted, spread with ½ cup cottage cheese and topped with 5 cherry tomatoes, halved, and 1 Tbsp. chopped chives and drizzled with olive oil, served with coffee and half-and-half
(133 SUGAR CALORIES, not 407 Calories)

1 fried egg on top of a piece of buttered whole wheat toast, sprinkled with 2 Tbsp. Parmesan cheese and served with 2 Italian sausage links and coffee with half-and-half
(57 SUGAR CALORIES, not 703 Calories)

Lunch: 1 cup cooked penne pasta mixed with 3 cooked, chopped bacon strips, ¼ cup chopped kale, ¼ cup halved cherry tomatoes, ⅛ cup ranch dressing, all served on top of 3 halved Romaine lettuce leaves
(182 SUGAR CALORIES, not 504 Calories)

1 red bell pepper, cored and seeded filled with a mixture of ¼ cup black beans, ¼ cup rice, ½ sautéed chopped celery stalk, ¼ sautéed chopped onion, ½ sautéed minced garlic clove, ¼ cup spinach, ⅛ cup shredded pepper jack cheese, 1 tsp. cumin covered with aluminum foil and baked at 350 degrees for 1 hour
(87 SUGAR CALORIES, not 240 Calories)

Dinner: Bake a pizza using a whole wheat pita with 3 slices mozzarella, 4 pepperoni slices, 1 Tbsp. chopped onion, 1 Tbsp. chopped green bell pepper, and 2 Tbsp. black olives, served with 1 cup salad mix with 5 cherry tomatoes, 1 Tbsp. Parmesan, and 3 Tbsp. blue cheese dressing
(95 SUGAR CALORIES, not 678 Calories)

3 sautéed scallops served over ½ cup mashed potatoes, topped with 1 Tbsp. melted butter, 1 Tbsp. chopped chives, and salt and pepper to taste
(71 SUGAR CALORIES, not 316 CALORIES)

*Note: For tracking your Sugar Calories—if you are eating a food that is not on the provided food lists look at the label and determine the amount of Sugar Calories by multiplying the carb grams on the label by 4.

Conclusion

With The 100™ Plus or the Weekend Plan you'll be set to eat anywhere to match any mood or occasion. Turn to the next chapter for extensive food lists that will give you a multitude of options. Happy eating!

8

The Food Lists

Currently the USDA has Recommended Daily
Allowance of 1,752 SUGAR CALORIES or
around 9 cups of sugar.

The things I wish were true:

■ If no one sees you eat it, it has no calories.

■ If you drink a diet soda with candy, they cancel each other out.

■ Foods used for medicinal purposes have no calories. This includes any chocolate used for energy, Sara Lee cheesecake (eaten whole), and Häagen-Dazs ice cream.

■ Movie-related foods are much lower in calories simply because they are a part of the entertainment experience and not part of one's personal fuel. This includes (but is not limited to) Milk Duds, popcorn with butter, Junior Mints, Snickers, and Gummi Bears.

■ If you eat the food off someone else's plate, it doesn't count.

■ If you eat standing up, the calories all go to your feet and get walked off.

■ Food eaten at Christmas parties has 0 calories, courtesy of Santa.

The foods that are lowest in Sugar Calories are the foods that will super-charge your weight loss because they keep insulin at low levels, which means you can burn fat at higher rates for more hours of each day. These are the foods that will be the foundation of your daily eating plan, and this is how all the menus are set up. This strategy also keeps you from having uncontrollable cravings that can sabotage your efforts. Remember, when insulin is spiked, as it is with highly refined, easily digestible sugars and starches, it causes your body to store its fuel as fat, it makes you hungrier faster than low-insulin foods will, and it causes cravings for more of the same unhealthy foods.

The following lists are a shortcut to my calculations for many common foods. If you are counting the Sugar Calories yourself, you simply need to mul-tiply the number of carbohydrate grams on any food label by 4. In the case that you are eating out or at a coffee bar where just the full calorie count is provided, I suggest that you count the full calories toward your Sugar Calories, so you are sure to stay within 100 calories per day. Since virtually all nutrition labels are available online, you can always figure out the carbohydrate grams and calcu-late your Sugar Calories for any food later in the day.

The way it works is simple: You have 100 Sugar Calories a day to choose from and you can use them anyway you like.

These foods don't need to be counted, just refer back to chapter 3 on page 91 for the portion suggestions, and create the meals that appeal to you.

Proteins—0 SUGAR CALORIES

Poultry

Chicken breast

Cornish hen

Lean ground turkey

Turkey breast

Eggs

Chicken (brown or white)

Duck

Egg whites

Goose

Fish & Seafood

Catfish

Clams

Cod

Crab

Flounder

Halibut

Lobster

Mahimahi

Orange roughy

Oysters

Salmon

Sardines

Scallops

Shrimp

Sole

Swordfish

Tilapia

Trout

Tuna

Beef, Pork, Veal, Lamb

Select or Choice grades of beef trimmed of fat including: chuck, rib, rump roast, round, sirloin, cubed, flank, porterhouse, T-bone steak, tenderloin

Bacon

Beef jerky

Canadian bacon

Ground beef

Ham

Lamb chop, leg, or roast

Pork center loin chop

Pork tenderloin

Veal loin, chop, or roast

Other Proteins

Bierwurst or beerwurst

Bologna

Buffalo

Chorizo

Corned beef

Devon (sausage)

Duck

Goose

Ham

Hot dog

Jay Robb Whey Protein

Liverwurst

Meatloaf—Pastrami

Pepperoni—Smoked meat

Pheasant

Pork roll

Processed sandwich/deli meats (ham, roast beef, turkey, chicken, etc.)

Prosciutto

Roast beef

Roast pork

Salami—Capicola

Sausage

Summer sausage

Turkey bacon

Turkey burger

Vegetarian Meats

Chik'n Strips, Meal Starter, MorningStar Farms

Hot dogs, Smart Dogs, Lightlife

Tofu

Veggie burgers, Garden Veggie Patties, MorningStar Farms

Vegetables—0 SUGAR CALORIES

Alfalfa spouts

Artichokes

Arugula

Asparagus

Bell pepper, red

Bok choy, regular or baby

Broccoli

Brussels sprouts

Cabbage

Cauliflower

Celery

Chard, Swiss

Collards

Corn, white

Cucumber

Eggplant

Endive

Fennel

Green onion

Kale

Lettuce, iceberg

Lettuce, red leaf

Lettuce, Romaine

Mushrooms

Mustard greens

Okra

Pepper, jalapeño

Pepper, serrano

Pickles, dill

Radicchio

Radishes

Scallions

Seaweed

Shallots

Snap peas

Spinach

Summer squash

Turnip greens

Watercress

Zucchini

Herbs & Spices—0 SUGAR CALORIES

Basil, fresh

Chives

Cilantro

Garlic

Ginger

Parsley

Pepper

Peppermint, fresh

Salt

Thyme, fresh

Fats—0 SUGAR CALORIES

Animal Fats

Avocado Oil

Barlean's Coconut Oil

Barlean's Flaxseed oil

Barlean's Omega Swirl Flax Oil (multiple flavors: Lemon, Strawberry
Banana, Orange Cream, Pomegranate Blueberry, Chocolate
Raspberry)

Butter

Ghee

Olive Oil

Saturated Fats

Sesame Oil

Walnut Oil

Dairy Products—0 SUGAR CALORIES

Cheese

American

Asiago

Blue

Brick

Brie

Cheddar

Colby

Colby jack

Cottage cheese

Dry jack

Edam

Farmer cheese

Feta

Fontina

Gorgonzola

Gouda

Gruyère

Havarti

Limburger

Mascarpone

Monterey jack

Mozzarella

Muenster

Parmesan

Pepato

Pepper jack

Provolone

Queso blanco

Ricotta

Romano

Scamorza

Soy cheese

Swiss

Teleme

Other

Almond milk, unsweetened

Coconut milk, unsweetened

FAGE Total Greek Yogurt

Half-and-half

Sour cream

Soy milk, unsweetened

Whipped cream

Other—0 SUGAR CALORIES

Almond flour

Almonds

Avocado

Baking powder

Baking soda

Barlean's Forti-Flax

Brazil nuts

Cashews

Coffee, black

Espresso

Lemon

Lime

Macadamia nuts

Mayonnaise

Mustard

Onion

Pine nuts

Powdered mix, Stevia Tropical Singles

Pumpkin seeds

Sesame seeds

Soy sauce

Sparkling water

Sunflower seeds

Tea, unsweetened plain, hot or iced

Tomato

Vinegar

Water

THE 100 | Sugar Calories

I have created a list of many common foods that are important to count toward your daily allowance of 100 Sugar Calories. If a food is not listed below, but is not on the Freebie list, make sure to look up the Total Carbohydrate amount and multiply by 4 to get the Sugar Calorie total.

Dairy Products

Milk, 1% or fat free (1 cup) = 49 SUGAR CALORIES

Milk, whole (1 cup) = 51 SUGAR CALORIES

Nonfat dry milk (⅓ cup) = 12 SUGAR CALORIES

Rice milk, plain, Rice Dream (1 cup) = 92 SUGAR CALORIES

Soy milk, plain, Silk (1 cup) = 32 SUGAR CALORIES

Yogurt, fat-free, plain (6 oz) = 52 SUGAR CALORIES

Legumes

Black beans, cooked (½ cup) = 92 SUGAR CALORIES

Baked beans, original, Bush Brothers (¼ cup) = 116 SUGAR CALORIES

Chickpeas/garbanzo beans (½ cup) = 65 SUGAR CALORIES

Edamame (shelled soybeans) (½ cup) = 40 SUGAR CALORIES

Green beans (1 cup) = 32 SUGAR CALORIES

Hummus (2 Tbsp.) = 16 SUGAR CALORIES

Kidney beans (¼ cup) = 40 SUGAR CALORIES

Lentils (¼ cup) = 40 SUGAR CALORIES

Pinto beans (¼ cup) = 44 SUGAR CALORIES

Carbohydrates

Breads and Tortillas

Bagels, honey whole wheat (1) = 224 SUGAR CALORIES

Bread, sprouted whole grain (1 slice) = 60 SUGAR CALORIES

Bread, whole wheat (1 slice) = 88 SUGAR CALORIES

Hamburger bun (1) = 72 SUGAR CALORIES

Hamburger bun, sprouted whole grain (1) = 136 SUGAR CALORIES

Pancake, plain frozen, ready-to-heat (4" diameter, 1) = 60 SUGAR CALORIES

Pita, whole wheat (1) = 62 SUGAR CALORIES

Roll, small dinner (1) = 52 SUGAR CALORIES

Tortilla, corn (6" diameter, 1) = 23 SUGAR CALORIES

Tortilla, flour (6" diameter, 1) = 64 SUGAR CALORIES

Wrap, organic whole wheat (1) = 80 SUGAR CALORIES

Waffle, frozen, ready-to-heat (4" diameter, 1) = 60 SUGAR CALORIES

Pasta

Penne, whole wheat, cooked (1 cup) = 208 SUGAR CALORIES

Spaghetti, whole wheat, cooked (1 cup) = 151 SUGAR CALORIES

Spirals, whole wheat, cooked (1 cup) = 149 SUGAR CALORIES

Cereals and Grains

Basmati rice, cooked (½ cup) = 88 SUGAR CALORIES

Brown rice, cooked (½ cup) = 92 SUGAR CALORIES

Cereal, dry, Cheerios (¾ cup) = 72 SUGAR CALORIES

Cereal, dry, shredded wheat, Post (1 cup) = 164 SUGAR CALORIES

Cereal, dry, Uncle Sam's (¾ cup) = 152 SUGAR CALORIES

Cereal, dry, Total (¾ cup) = 92 SUGAR CALORIES

Cereal, dry, Wheaties (¾ cup) = 88 SUGAR CALORIES

Cereal, dry, whole grain ground flax, Ezekiel 4:9 (¾ cup) = 222 SUGAR CALORIES

Cereal, dry whole grain, Ezekiel 4:9 (½ cup) = 160 SUGAR CALORIES

Couscous, cooked (½ cup) = 73 SUGAR CALORIES

Corn muffin mix, "Jiffy" (¼ cup) = 108 SUGAR CALORIES

Granola, low-fat (½ cup) = 160 SUGAR CALORIES

Jasmine rice, cooked (½ cup) = 106 SUGAR CALORIES

Oatmeal, dry steel cut (¼ cup) = 108 SUGAR CALORIES

Oatmeal, original instant, Quaker (1 packet) = 76 SUGAR CALORIES

Oatmeal, instant apples and cinnamon, Quaker (1 packet) = 88 SUGAR CALORIES

Spanish rice, cooked (½ cup) = 80 SUGAR CALORIES

Quinoa, cooked (½ cup) = 79 SUGAR CALORIES

White rice, cooked (½ cup) = 106 SUGAR CALORIES

Vegetables

Turnip, cubes (1 cup) = 34 SUGAR CALORIES

Vegetable blend, stir fry frozen (¾ cup) = 20 SUGAR CALORIES

Corn, yellow (½ cup) = 58 SUGAR CALORIES

French fries, fast food (1 large) = 260 SUGAR CALORIES

Potato (1 medium) = 146 SUGAR CALORIES

Winter squash, acorn (½ cup) = 75 SUGAR CALORIES

Winter squash, butternut (½ cup) = 43 SUGAR CALORIES

Rutabaga, cubes (1 cup) = 58 SUGAR CALORIES

Yam (½ cup) = 75 SUGAR CALORIES

Sweet potato (1 medium) = 92 SUGAR CALORIES

Fruits

Fruits are healthy and have lots of vitamins—but they are primarily carbohydrates and natural sugar, so we do need to pay attention to calories because they spike insulin. The jury is out on these foods; some agencies and experts say that the sugar and carbs in fruit do not count because they are offset by fiber and water content, but others say that it can still alter weight loss. Based on this I suggest keeping fruit servings to no more than 2 per day.

Apple (1 medium) = 99 SUGAR CALORIES

Apricot (1 medium) = 16 SUGAR CALORIES

Banana (1 medium) = 108 SUGAR CALORIES

Blackberries (½ cup) = 29 SUGAR CALORIES

Blueberries (½ cup) = 43 SUGAR CALORIES

Cantaloupe (1 wedge) = 19 SUGAR CALORIES

Cherries (9) = 47 SUGAR CALORIES

Dried bananas (¼ cup) = 240 SUGAR CALORIES

Honeydew (1 wedge) = 46 SUGAR CALORIES

Kiwi (1 medium) = 40 SUGAR CALORIES

Mango, sliced (½ cup) = 52 SUGAR CALORIES

Oranges (1 small) = 45 SUGAR CALORIES

Peach (1 medium) = 59 SUGAR CALORIES

Pear (1 small) = 92 SUGAR CALORIES

Pineapple, diced (½ cup) = 43 SUGAR CALORIES

Plum (1 medium) = 30 SUGAR CALORIES

Raspberries (1 cup) = 59 SUGAR CALORIES

Red and pink grapefruit (½) = 21 SUGAR CALORIES

Strawberries (½ cup) = 26 SUGAR CALORIES

Tangerines (1 medium) = 47 SUGAR CALORIES

Watermelon, diced (1 cup) = 46 SUGAR CALORIES

Snacks & Treats

Cheese puffs, jumbo, Cheetos (1 oz) = 60 SUGAR CALORIES

Chips, lightly salted, Kettle (1 oz) = 76 SUGAR CALORIES

Chips, nacho cheese, Doritos (1 oz) = 68 SUGAR CALORIES

Chips, original, Popchips (22 chips) = 80 SUGAR CALORIES

Chocolate, Intense Dark 86% Cacao Ghiardelli (4 pieces) =
   60 SUGAR CALORIES

Chocolate, organic dark 85% Green and Black's (12 pieces) =
   60 SUGAR CALORIES

Cookies, chocolate chip or oatmeal, Joseph's (4 cookies) =
   52 SUGAR CALORIES

Cookies, chocolate crème cookies, Newman's Own (2 cookies) =
   80 SUGAR CALORIES

Corn snack, Pirate's Booty (1 oz) = 72 SUGAR CALORIES

Crackers, goldfish, Pepperidge Farms (55 pieces) = 80 SUGAR
   CALORIES

Crackers, Nabisco Ritz Original (5) = 40 SUGAR CALORIES

Crackers, multigrain, Nabisco Wheat Thins (6) = 88 SUGAR
   CALORIES

Crispbread, Wasa Original (2 pieces) = 80 SUGAR CALORIES

Granola bars, oats, fruits & nuts (1 bar) = 88 SUGAR CALORIES

Ice cream, soft serve, vanilla (½ cup) = 70 SUGAR CALORIES

Kettle corn (1 cup) = 100 SUGAR CALORIES

Popcorn, air popped (3 cups) = 75 SUGAR CALORIES

Rice cakes, lightly salted, Quaker (2) = 56 SUGAR CALORIES

Trail mix (1 oz) = 45 SUGAR CALORIES

Beverages

Beer, non-alcoholic, O'Doul's (1 bottle) = 53 SUGAR CALORIES

Soda, organic sparkling green tea, Steaz (1 can) = 92 SUGAR CALORIES

Apple juice (8 oz) = 116 SUGAR CALORIES

Beer, Michelob Ultra (1 bottle) = 10 SUGAR CALORIES

Beer, Miller Lite (1 bottle) = 13 SUGAR CALORIES

Beer, Coors Light (1 bottle) = 20 SUGAR CALORIES

Cola, Diet Coke (8 oz) = 0 SUGAR CALORIES (contains artificial sweeteners)

Energy drink, Diet Rockstar (8 oz) = 8 SUGAR CALORIES (contains artificial sweeteners)

Energy drink, sugar free, Red Bull (8 oz) = 11 SUGAR CALORIES (contains artificial sweeteners)

Sports drink, Gatorade, lemonade (4 oz) = 30 SUGAR CALORIES

Ginger ale, Schweppes (4 oz) = 46 SUGAR CALORIES

Grapefruit juice, light, Ocean Spray (8 oz) = 120 SUGAR CALORIES

Vegetable juice, V8 100% (8 oz) = 40 SUGAR CALORIES

Wine, white (1 glass, 3 oz) = 15 SUGAR CALORIES

Wine, dessert (1 glass, 3 oz) = 80 SUGAR CALORIES

Wine, red (1 glass, 3 oz) = 14 SUGAR CALORIES

Condiments & Dressings

Almond butter (2 Tbsp.) = 27 SUGAR CALORIES

Hot sauce (1 Tbsp.) = 1 SUGAR CALORIE

Italian dressing (2 Tbsp.) = 12 SUGAR CALORIES

Ketchup (1 Tbsp.) = 15 SUGAR CALORIES

Miracle Whip, light, Kraft (2 Tbsp.) = 24 SUGAR CALORIES

Natural sweetener, Stevia powder (1 packet) = 4 SUGAR CALORIES

Natural sweetener, Xylitol Crystals (1 Tbsp.) = 24 SUGAR
CALORIES

Peanut butter (2 Tbsp.) = 25 SUGAR CALORIES

Ranch dressing (2 Tbsp.) = 8 SUGAR CALORIES

Salsa (2 Tbsp.) = 8 SUGAR CALORIES

Apple sauce, unsweetened (½ cup) = 56 SUGAR CALORIES

Cocktail sauce (⅛ cup) = 30 SUGAR CALORIES

Honey (1 Tbsp.) = 69 SUGAR CALORIES

Barbecue sauce (2 Tbsp.) = 102 SUGAR CALORIES

Teriyaki, ready-to-serve (2 Tbsp.) = 28 SUGAR CALORIES

Frozen Foods

Amy's, Frozen Meals (1)

Black Bean and Vegetable Enchilada = 88 SUGAR CALORIES

Shepherd's Pie = 108 SUGAR CALORIES

Spinach Feta Pocket Sandwich = 136 SUGAR CALORIES

Mexican Tofu Scramble = 160 SUGAR CALORIES

Lean Cuisine, Frozen Meals (1)

Alfredo Pasta with Chicken & Broccoli = 180 SUGAR CALORIES

Baked Chicken = 120 SUGAR CALORIES

Beef Pot Roast = 104 SUGAR CALORIES

Chicken and Vegetables = 116 SUGAR CALORIES

Chicken Marsala = 116 SUGAR CALORIES

Garlic Beef and Broccoli = 172 SUGAR CALORIES

Glazed Chicken = 116 SUGAR CALORIES

Grilled Chicken Caesar Bowl = 132 SUGAR CALORIES

Lemongrass Chicken = 140 SUGAR CALORIES

Meatloaf with Gravy & Whipped Potatoes = 100 SUGAR
CALORIES

Roasted Chicken with Lemon Pepper Fettuccini = 112 SUGAR
CALORIES

Roasted Garlic Chicken = 44 SUGAR CALORIES

Roasted Turkey & Vegetables = 72 SUGAR CALORIES

Rosemary Chicken = 108 SUGAR CALORIES

Salmon with Basil = 100 SUGAR CALORIES

Salisbury Steak with Mac & Cheese = 92 SUGAR CALORIES

Shrimp Alfredo = 112 SUGAR CALORIES

Shrimp and Angel Hair Pasta = 136 SUGAR CALORIES

Steak Tips Portobello = 56 SUGAR CALORIES

Stuffed Cabbage = 112 SUGAR CALORIES

Swedish Meatballs = 140 SUGAR CALORIES

JORGE: Gary, this is something I have to ask. Everybody asks me about fruit. If you are a woman or a man and you are just trying to lose weight, we all love the fruits and sweets, things like that. If there were some fruits for women what are the ones that are good for weight loss?

GARY: I don't think any of them cause weight loss.

JORGE: Because most fruits have—drum roll.

GARY: They have sugar and glucose.

JORGE: A lot of people say those are natural sugars. Those don't count.

GARY: It is not a question of whether they count or not. The problem is once we are fat we must keep our insulin levels low—like we said, the biology tells us we want the insulin levels to be as low as possible.

JORGE: Which means all sugars? Natural included?

GARY: Any. You know you have to get rid of all refined grains, but arguably berries, blueberries, are fine.

THE 100 | Conclusion

Congratulations, you are now equipped with a full list of foods to pick from when you are feeling adventurous. With this knowledge in hand you are ready to start putting together meals on your own and maybe, if you are so bold, start creating your own recipes. Good job!

KATIE

VITAL STATS

AGE: 41   **HEIGHT:** 5' 6"   **WEIGHT LOST:** 54 pounds

MY BEST STRATEGY: Embrace this way of life. When I first started eating in this new way, I was skeptical. It was so different from everything I'd ever heard about eating healthy and losing weight, but after I lost 12 pounds in the first week, I was sold. I love that I'm never hungry with this system, because I'd never before been able to lose weight and not feel hungry. I follow this program to the letter and it's brought me huge success.

When I was younger, I was the classic pear shape, and I always packed on extra weight in my hips and thighs, but as I hit my fourth decade of life, the weight started to go to my belly. I knew that becoming an "apple" was more dangerous for my heart and health and it helped me become motivated to make a change. Finding this way of eating was a real breakthrough that allowed me to shed the pounds and to keep them off for good. This plan is so simple to follow, and it really works, plus it's a way of eating that I can truly be happy with. I never have to think about cheating because I can always have whatever I want.

Forget to Exercise

> When surveying the scientific literature on the
> treatment of obesity one cannot help but come
> away . . . underwhelmed by the minor contribution
> of exercise to most weight-loss programs.
> —JUDITH STERN, NUTRITIONIST AND OBESITY
> EXPERT AT THE UNIVERSITY OF CALIFORNIA, DAVIS.

A book about weight loss without a fitness routine? I know it's unheard of, and I'm not saying that exercise isn't good for a variety of things—it improves overall fitness, banishes the blues, increases your cognitive abilities (clearer thinking, ability to focus, improved memory), ramps up your immune system to fight disease, decreases back and body pain, and lowers heart disease risk—but one thing that exercise isn't effective at is helping you to lose weight.

THE 100 | Exercise Won't Help You Lose Weight

There. I said it. I know we hear it all the time—if you want to get slim, you'd better exercise—but the science doesn't back it up. And when you take a closer look at the recommendations from many of our government and health agencies you can see that they really aren't promising weight loss for your time on the treadmill.

The USDA The dietary guidelines of the U.S. Department of Agriculture recommend that we engage in up to 60 minutes of moderate to vigorous exercise on a daily basis just to maintain weight.

The AHA and the ACSM The American Heart Association and the American College of Sports Medicine published joint guidelines for exercise that suggest 30 minutes of moderate physical activity 5 days a week to promote and maintain health.

The IOM The Institute of Medicine of the National Academies also recommends 60 minutes a day of exercise to avoid weight gain.

The International Association for the Study of Obesity This association dittos the USDA and the IOM recommendation for an hour of exercise a day to avoid gaining weight as well.

The WHO The World Health Organization recommends 150 minutes a week (30 minutes, 5 days a week) of moderate physical activity for all adults. The benefits included in exercise according to the WHO are:

lower rates of death, heart disease, high blood pressure, stroke, type 2 diabetes, metabolic syndrome, colon and breast cancer, and depression;

likely to have less risk of a hip or vertebral fracture;

exhibit a higher level of cardiorespiratory and muscular fitness; and

are more likely to achieve weight maintenance, have a healthier body
mass and composition.

What none of these agencies say is that physical activity will lead to weight loss.

These authorities on health often cite a Finnish review that was published in 2000. The researchers analyzed data of all the relevant research on exercise and weight loss for the past two decades—this study is considered the most rigorous scientific evidence to date—but it doesn't really prove that exercise helps with weight loss. In the end, all dieters in all studies appeared to regain the weight they'd lost despite efforts to exercise. What exercise seemed to do was either delay the rate of regain by small amounts (3.2 ounces per month) or increase it (1.8 ounces per month).

Why Is Exercise Recommended for Weight Loss?

Fact: Lean people are more physically active than fat people. But this doesn't mean that exercise causes thinness any more than sedentary behavior causes fatness. A fat person won't become thin because they exercise, and a thin person won't get fat if they stop exercising. The problem is that many obesity experts, nutritionists, and personal trainers use a simple math theory that if you just cut the right amount of calories (to create a calorie deficit) then you will lose weight. This comes from the old calories in/calories out theory. The equation is correct, and it goes like this: 3100 calories is equal to 1 pound of fat, so to lose one pound of fat in one week you simply need to cut calories and burn more—specifically 100 calories a day minus your resting metabolism rate. Many weight loss recommendations suggest a combination of diet and exercise to do this, it seems simple right? Just cut 200 calories a day from your diet, and exercise off 300 calories. Unfortunately, this doesn't often work out to add up to the weight loss people so desire.

Why Exercise Won't Cause Weight Loss

The biggest reason working out fails to produce weight loss is that exercise makes us hungrier, and, in the end, we clever humans either eat more, or we find a way to conserve energy. So basically, we compensate. Remember homeostasis in chapter 2? Our bodies always work to maintain balance. This includes calories and weight. If you burn more calories, the odds are good that you'll eat more the same day, or the next day—in the end, your body will work hard to make sure that you maintain your weight. Gary Taubes, my mentor, and author of *Good Calories, Bad Calories,* writes, "When we are physically active, we work up an appetite. Hunger increases in proportion to the calories we expend, just as restricting the calories in our diet will leave us hungry until we eventually make good the deficit, if not more." When Danish researchers trained nonathletes to run a marathon (18 men, 9 women) over 18 months they found that the men lost an average of 5 pounds of body fat, while the women stayed exactly the same weight. "The importance of exercise in weight control is less than might be believed, because increases in energy expenditure due to exercise also tend to increase food consumption, and it is not possible to predict whether the increased caloric output will be outweighed by the greater food intake," concluded a report put forth from a 1979 National Institutes of Health Conference.

Interestingly, until the 1960s, doctors who treated the overweight and obese didn't recommend exercise. In fact, no one believed that exercise would help you lose weight at that time. Experts felt that exercise slowed the rate of weight loss because it burns an insignificant number of calories but still increases your appetite. Even Louis Newburgh, the father of the calories in/calories out equation, calculated that these efforts were futile for weight loss. In 1942, Newburgh figured that a 250-pound man would only burn three calories climbing a flight of stairs—not even half a teaspoon of sugar and he'd be back to square one. That same man would have to climb 20 flights to eat an apple and call it even, not a very realistic endeavor, so Newburgh concluded that exercise wasn't worth it.

So, why do so many of us have gym memberships, running shoes, and dumbbells in our possession today? Our exercise explosion came about in the early 1970s when a new conventional wisdom was born that exercise is good for you. By 1980, one hundred million Americans were exercising regularly according to the *Washington Post*. From 1972 to 2005, gyms reported that revenues increased from 200 million to 16 billion dollars. And marathon numbers have increased from 300 participants per various marathons in the 1960s to more than 39,000 in 2008. The reason this started happening, as with the low-fat craze, is because of research—faulty research, it turns out—that indicated that exercise could cause this calorie deficit and that some evidence found that it didn't cause hunger. However, the research that was done boiled down to two studies, one with rats, and one with humans in India, and these studies did support the idea just stated, but no other researcher (and many have tried) has ever been able to replicate these studies. So we have two studies that say, yes, you can exercise to lose weight, and probably a hundred or more that say, no, it doesn't work. I'm betting on the multiple, more rigorous, and more recent scientific research.

The bottom line—disregarding the research—is that we exercise way more today than we did in the 1960s—and we are burning many more calories through physical activity than we used to—so then, why do the rates of obesity continue to climb with all this added activity? Exercise obviously isn't working because it either causes us to eat too much, or to conserve energy after a workout. The answer is in what we discussed in the previous chapters—ultimately our obesity epidemic is due to the overconsumption of highly refined, easily digestible carbohydrates and sugars, which chronically elevates insulin, which, in turn, tells our bodies to store food as fat, and not use it as fuel.

That's why I made the decision to forgo another chapter with a fitness routine outlined in it. That said, I still think it is a great idea to include enjoyable levels of exercise for the reasons mentioned in the beginning of this chapter.

Take a bike ride on a sunny day to improve your mood, go for a walk with a friend and lower your blood pressure, lift weights at the gym to improve your muscle tone, take an aerobics class to improve your lung capacity and lower your risk of heart disease—just don't expect your exercise to aid your weight loss. For successful weight loss, follow The 100™.

THE 100 | An Exercise Routine That Can Improve Appearance

If you are looking to decrease flabbiness and increase fitness and muscle tone, it is far better to spend less time on the treadmill and more time lifting weights or doing sit-ups and push-ups. The great part about doing strength training is that you will build muscle, which will make your body look and feel more toned and trim.

After you've followed The 100™ for a couple weeks and feel you have adjusted to the new way of eating, consider giving the following workout a try. It should take you about 20 minutes, and you can do it up to 3 times a week, on nonconsecutive days.

The Workout

Do one set of 8 to 12 repetitions, and then immediately do one set of 8 to 12 reps of the next exercise, continue until all moves have been completed. If you can do an exercise more than 12 times, the weight is too light. If you can't reach 12 repetitions, the weight is too heavy.

Dumbbell Press

Lie on a mat on your back with your knees bent and your feet flat on the floor. You may place one or more pillows under your back and head for support. Holding a dumbbell in each hand, bring your elbows in line with your shoulders, making a right angle between your upper arm and your side. Exhale as you extend your arms and press the dumbbells toward the ceiling. Keep your elbows loose. Hold for 1 second. Inhale as you return to the starting point.

Row

Sit in a chair, and grasp a dumbbell in each hand. You may put a pillow on your lap for support. Lean forward, and extend your arms straight down, being sure to keep your elbows loose. Exhale as you slowly bring your elbows toward the ceiling. Once the dumbbells reach the top of your thighs, hold for 1 second. Inhale as you slowly lower the dumbbells.

Lateral Raises

Stand with your feet shoulder-width apart, your back straight, and your abs tight. Hold a dumbbell in each hand at your sides with your arms straight and your elbows loose. Exhale as you slowly lift the dumbbells out to the side until they are slightly above shoulder level and your palms are facing the floor. Hold for 1 second. Inhale as you lower your arms.

Crunches

Lie on a mat on your back with your knees bent and your feet flat on the floor. Make a fist with your right hand, and place it between your chin and collarbone. With your left hand, grasp your right wrist. This will prevent you from leading with your head and straining your neck. Without moving your lower body, exhale, and slowly curl your upper torso until your shoulder blades are off the floor. Hold for 1 second. Inhale as you slowly lower yourself.

Lying Triceps

Lie on a mat on your back with a dumbbell in each hand by your ears and the dumbbells pointing toward the ceiling. Straighten your arms, but keep your elbows loose. Hold for 1 second. Inhale as you return to the starting point.

Shoulder Curl

Stand with your feet shoulder-width apart. Hold a dumbbell in each hand at your sides with your arms extended. Exhale as you simultaneously curl both arms to just past 90 degrees, bringing your palms toward your biceps. Keep your elbows close to your sides, and concentrate on moving only from your elbow joints, not from your shoulders. Hold for 1 second. Inhale as you lower.

Squats

Stand with your feet slightly wider than shoulder-width apart. Keeping your back straight and your abs tight, exhale as you slowly squat down to about 90 degrees. Don't let your knees extend past your toes. Make sure to push your butt out as if you were sitting in a chair. Hold for 1 second. Inhale as you slowly return to the starting position.

Exercise may not be the answer to losing weight, but it is still a valuable addition to your lifestyle. Not only will it reduce the jiggle in your wiggle by firming up flab, it can increase your lung capacity, improve insulin sensitivity, and keep your metabolism revved. The goal is to choose exercise you enjoy, not exercise that feels like a punishment. Consider activities that involve the whole family, such as bike rides, hiking, or swimming. If you're on your own, try a stress-relieving activity such as yoga or tai chi, or a fun social activity like Zumba or kickboxing.

Now, go have fun!

"I DID IT!"

BRENDA

VITAL STATS

AGE: 36   **HEIGHT:** 5' 8"   **WEIGHT LOST:** 15 pounds

MY BEST STRATEGY: Have a support system or a weight-loss buddy. For me it is my husband who was willing to change his eating habits along with mine. It's been great to have a loving teammate who wants to learn about new ways of eating healthy, cooking, and shopping together. We cheer each other on through tough times, and look for healthy activities such as hiking or biking together on the weekends. Being on this weight-loss journey together has transformed our marriage.

I used to suffer from migraines, back pain, and neck pain that were so bad I had to be on medications. Being able to lose the weight has helped me have more energy to be active, and the pain has gone away. I know that it's the result of not eating the processed or highly refined foods I used to eat that has done away with my migraines, and losing the weight has helped ease my back and neck pain. On top of the health benefits, I love how I look today. It makes me feel like a teenager again.

APPENDIX I

Comparing and Contrasting Popular Diets

The problem with most popular diets, as discussed in chapter 2, is that they tend to treat all calories as equals, and to view the path to weight loss as achievable only through cutting back on calories, and expending more than you consume. The problem with this strategy is that you are left so hungry that you can't maintain this way of eating, your metabolism plummets (your body's calorie burning engine slows down), and these diets keep Sugar Calories at too high a level, which keeps your blood sugar spiked, and your insulin elevated. In the end, you are following a diet that sets you up to fail because it inherently uses a strategy that causes your body to hold on to fat and to even increase more fat into your fat cells.

To illustrate the difference between some of the most popular diets—specifically Weight Watchers, Nutrisystem, Jenny Craig, and the Mayo Clinic Diet—on the market, I've included a comparison, and commentary on each. Warning: This information is for the detail oriented, meaning that I've included far more information than is necessary for succeeding at following The 100™. That said, I believe that looking at this information illuminates just how other diets miss the mark by providing far too many hidden and insulin-spiking Sugar Calories.

Here you'll find a sample one day menu for each of the four diets mentioned above, as well as one for The 100™. These charts show how each diet adds up if you calculate for Sugar Calories. Remember that these are the calories that spike blood sugar, trigger insulin, and causes your body to gain and store body and belly fat. Since many of these diets include packaged food, I calculated the Sugar Calories from the carbohydrate grams on the nutrient labels provided. There may indeed be some Freebie food components to these packaged foods, but that's the problem with packaged, processed foods—it's hard to separate the good from the bad. Better to eat real foods.

THE 100 | Comparing and Contrasting Popular Diets

Before I show you the entire days' eats for each diet, take a look at the total Sugar Calories for each diet (below).

Calculating Sugar Calories Remember that Sugar Calories are the carb grams per serving of food you are eating multiplied by 4 (1 gram of carbohydrate = 4 calories). Just by looking at these totals you can easily see how the calorie-restricted, low-fat diets—which Nutrisystem, Jenny Craig, Weight Watchers, and the Mayo Clinic Diet are—give you too many Sugar Calories per day even though they restrict overall calories, and therefore spike your insulin to a level that will sabotage your weight loss.

Total Calories While total calorie counts are not included below—because, as we discussed, it is not total calories that count, but the Sugar Calories in carbohydrates—do know that all diets come in at between 1,400 and 1,600 total calories per day.

Totals for each diet at a glance

NUTRISYSTEM		
	Carb Grams	Sugar Calories (rounded)
Totals per day	174.4	698

JENNY CRAIG		
	Carb Grams	Sugar Calories
Totals per day	234	936

THE MAYO CLINIC DIET		
	Carb Grams	Sugar Calories
Totals per day	222.4	890

WEIGHT WATCHERS		
	Carb Grams	Sugar Calories
Totals per day	191.2	764

THE 100		
	Carb Grams	Sugar Calories
Totals per day	23.694	356

Now let's take a closer look at each individual diet and the details for sugars, carbs, total calories, and Sugar Calories.

Nutrisystem

This diet is touted as one for those who are looking for the ultimate in convenience. On their website, you pick a month's worth of three meals per day plus one snack or dessert. The real foods added are 3 large servings of fruit, and 3 small servings of proteins or dairy choices, and 2 small servings of fat. Below is how a typical day would look. I chose the foods that were the most popular among clients to design a realistic day for a Nutrisystem client.

Most notably, the Nutrisystem model delivers a dangerous level of hidden sugars that are akin to drinking almost two cans of soda per day. At this level your body can't lose weight long-term because your blood sugar and insulin are so elevated that you will have cravings and hunger that will sabotage your efforts in the long run. Another issue is the number of overall calories, just over 1,300 calories, which makes this diet a member of the semi-starvation crew. You can't stay satisfied on this number of calories, especially when so many of these calories come from unsatisfying and hunger producing Sugar Calories. Earlier in this book, in chapter 2, I reviewed studies that looked at calorie-restricted diets, as you'll see with the other three diets below, these all fall into the range of calories, and the types of calories that leave subjects feeling weak, hungry, and miserable—and ultimately fail.

Nutrisystem

Meal: Breakfast	Total carbohydrate grams, or freebie	Sugar Calories (rounded)
NS Turkey Sausage & Egg Muffin	22	88
Blueberries, 1 cup	21.4	86
1 String Cheese	freebie	0
Meal: Lunch	**Total carbohydrate grams, or freebie**	**Sugar Calories**
NS Hamburger	28	112
Salad	freebie	0
Peanuts, 2 Tbsp.	freebie	0
Fat-free salad dressing, Italian, 2 Tbsp.	2.5	10
Meal: Snack	**Total carbohydrate grams, or freebie**	**Sugar Calories**
Apple, 1 medium	24.7	99
Nonfat milk, 1 cup	12.3	49
Meal: Dinner	**Total carbohydrate grams, or freebie**	**Sugar Calories**
NS Turkey and Italian Sausage Pizza	31	124
Broccoli and Asparagus	freebie	0
Strawberries, 1 cup	11	44
Olive Oil, 1 tsp.	freebie	0
Meal: Dessert	**Total carbohydrate grams, or freebie**	**Sugar Calories**
NS Walnut Chocolate Chip Cookies	17	68
Totals per day	**169.9**	**680**

Jenny Craig

This diet is another that falls under the convenience category because they allow you to order packaged foods, and supplement with small amounts of grocery items. Jenny Craig likes to tout the use of the volumetric theory of author Barbara Rolls, which says that your body will feel fuller by bulking up the volume of foods with liquids and whipping things up with air. But, in reality, this is just another low-calorie diet that has more than 900 Sugar Calories per day and a whopping 123 grams of sugar, almost a whole week's worth of sugar. This way of eating will set you up to crave sugary foods, and will leave you feeling hungry and feeling deprived.

Jenny Craig

Meal: Breakfast	Total carbohydrate grams, or freebie	Sugar Calories
Cranberry Almond Cereal	35	140
Nonfat milk, 1 cup	12.3	49
1 medium apple	24.7	99
Meal: Snack	**Total carbohydrate grams, or freebie**	**Sugar Calories**
Chocolate Chip Snack Bar	23	92
½ cup strawberries	6.4	26
Meal: Lunch	**Total carbohydrate grams, or freebie**	**Sugar Calories**
Chicken Stuffed Sandwich (diced chicken, broccoli, and cheese)	37	148
Garden Salad	freebie	0
1 packet Jenny Craig Balsamic Dressing	5	20
Meal: Snack	**Total carbohydrate grams, or freebie**	**Sugar Calories**
1 cup cantaloupe	13.7	55
¾ cup low fat cottage cheese	freebie	0
Meal: Dinner	**Total carbohydrate grams, or freebie**	**Sugar Calories**
Meatloaf with BBQ Sauce, and side of roasted potatoes, broccoli, and carrots	30	120
Zucchini, ½ cup	freebie	0
1 tsp. margarine	freebie	0
Meal: Dessert	**Total carbohydrate grams, or freebie**	**Sugar Calories**
1 cup nonfat milk	12.3	49
Jenny Craig Triple Chocolate Cheese Cake	30	120
Totals per day	229.4	918

Weight Watchers

Weight Watchers works by boiling down all foods into a points system: Foods that are higher in fats and simple carbs (sugars and refined carbs) are given higher points, while foods that are high in lean protein and fiber are given lower points. Fruits and vegetables are given 0 points, so you can eat as much as you want of either. To determine how many points you can have per day, Weight Watchers does a calculation based on your weight, age, height, and amount you are going to lose. After the math is done, you are given a daily number of points, 26 to 30 is average for most women per day. In addition, everyone gets a weekly allotment of points, 49 per week for women, which can be "spent" any way you'd like. Now, Weight Watchers doesn't just let you eat with wild abandon, and even though you could use all your points on chocolate and still be following the loose guidelines of the PowerPlus Points system, Weight Watchers does educate members to maximize "power foods," and suggests serving sizes for certain foods. Here's how they measure up.

Fruits and Veggies It is recommended that you eat 5 servings of these a day (9 if you weigh more than 350 pounds), but Weight Watchers doesn't tell you to focus on low-sugar vegetables like spinach, and since the point value for both fruits and vegetables is 0, people on the program can eat as much as they want of fruits (which can overload the system with sugar) and not have it count toward their daily food plan.

Lean Proteins Weight Watchers suggests that you eat 1 to 2 servings of the leanest cuts of meat, fish and poultry, or about 6 ounces per day. The range of points is wide here, for 4 ounces of steak you are looking at 10 points, 3 ounces of chicken breast is 4 points, while 3 ounces of tilapia is just 2 points.

Dairy 2 servings per day of low-fat, nonfat, or fat-free milk, yogurt and cheeses. Cheese is around 2 points per ounce of cheese, or cup of nonfat milk or yogurt.

Whole grains While Weight Watchers does encourage higher fiber types of grains and breads, it doesn't recommend a serving size. Points are usually 2 per slice of bread or ½ cup of rice.

Fats Weight Watchers recommends 2 teaspoons of healthy oils per day. Including olive oil, flax, or canola. These are usually 1 point per tsp.

Liquid The recommendation is to drink at least 6 nonalcoholic beverages per day (interestingly, it doesn't say that these need to be sugar free).

Alcohol Weight Watchers recommends that women have no more than one 4 ounce glass of wine per day.

Based on these guidelines I've put together a day's menu to take a look at the Sugar Calories—which are off the chart.

Weight Watchers

Meal: Breakfast (points)	Total carbohydrate grams, or freebie	Sugar Calories	Points
1 cup plain instant oatmeal	27.3	109	4
1 cup fat-free cottage cheese	freebie	0	3
1 cup diced apple	30.3	121	0
Meal: Snack (points)	**Total carbohydrate grams, or freebie**	**Sugar Calories**	**Points**
5 cups microwave popcorn (94% fat free)	20	80	3
Meal: Lunch (points)	**Total carbohydrate grams, or freebie**	**Sugar Calories**	**Points**
½ cup cooked regular pasta	17.7	71	2
Diced tomatoes and chopped spinach to equal 2 cups	freebie	0	0
⅛ cup feta cheese	freebie	0	1.5
½ cup canned chicken, 4 oz.	freebie	0	5
1 tsp. olive oil	freebie	0	1
Meal: Dinner (points)	**Total carbohydrate grams, or freebie**	**Sugar Calories**	**Points**
4 oz. lean steak (round or loin cuts with all visible fat removed)	freebie	0	5
2 cups salad (lettuce, tomatoes, etc.)	freebie	0	0
1 cup brown rice	45.8	183	5
2 Tbsp. fat-free italian dressing	2.6	10	1
1 tsp. butter	freebie	0	1
Meal: Dessert (points)	**Total carbohydrate grams, or freebie**	**Sugar Calories**	**Points**
1 cup strawberries, sliced	12.7	51	0
¼ cup low-fat granola	19.5	78	2
½ cup fat-free greek yogurt, plain	4.5	18	1.5
Totals per day	**180.4**	**721**	**35**

Mayo Clinic

This is another example of a diet that allows far too many sugar and carb grams—as you can see from the Sugar Calories coming in at more than eight times as much as I recommend you having in a day. Once again, while you might be taking in a restricted amount of overall calories, the components of these calories set you up to fail.

Mayo Clinic

Meal: Breakfast	Total Carbohydrate grams, or freebie	Sugar Calories (rounded)
1 small banana, 5" long	18.7	73
½ cup bran cereal	16.1	64
1 cup nonfat milk	12.3	49
Meal: Snack	**Total Carbohydrate grams, or freebie**	**Sugar Calories**
1 small pear	22.9	92
1 oz. Cheddar cheese	freebie	0
Meal: Lunch	**Total Carbohydrate grams, or freebie**	**Sugar Calories**
4 oz. turkey breast sliced	freebie	0
2 pieces whole wheat bread	24	96
1 Tbsp. low-fat mayonnaise	freebie	0
lettuce and tomato	freebie	0
1 small apple	21.1	84
Meal: Snack	**Total Carbohydrate grams, or freebie**	**Sugar Calories**
1 cup sliced strawberries	12.7	51
1 oz. (about 7) Triscuit Baked Whole Wheat Original	19	76
Meal: Dinner	**Total Carbohydrate grams, or freebie**	**Sugar Calories**
2 oz. beef tenderloin	freebie	0
2 small red potatoes (2" diameter)	54.1	216
1 tsp. margarine (trans fat free)	0	0
Fat-free salad dressing, Italian, 2 Tbsp.	2.5	10
Meal: Dessert	**Total Carbohydrate grams, or freebie**	**Sugar Calories**
⅓ cup lemon sherbet	16.6	67
Totals per day	**220**	**878**

The 100™

With this food plan, not only do you get a diet that is full of satisfying, nutritious, and slowly digesting proteins, healthy fats, and Freebie Vegetables, your sugar grams are nice and low to keep your insulin and blood sugar at reduced rates so that your body can let go of long-stored fat, and not add any new fat to its stores, which means you'll lose weight.

The 100™

Meal: Breakfast	Total carbohydrate grams, or freebie	Sugar Calories	Points
2 scrambled eggs	freebie	0	4
2 sausage patties	freebie	0	6
Meal: Snack	Total carbohydrate grams, or freebie	Sugar Calories	Points
1 string cheese	freebie	0	0
Meal: Lunch (open-faced turkey patty with Swiss)	Total carbohydrate grams, or freebie	Sugar Calories	Points
1 slice Food For Life Sprouted Grain Ezekiel 4:9 Bread	15	60	2
1 slice Swiss cheese, 1 oz.	freebie	0	2
Ground turkey patty, 3 oz. cooked, 85% lean	freebie	0	4
Lettuce, tomato	freebie	0	0
Mayonnaise, 1 Tbsp.	freebie	0	3
Meal: Snack	Total carbohydrate grams, or freebie	Sugar Calories	Points
11 almonds, dry roasted	freebie	0	2.5
Meal: Dinner (prosciutto and feta spinach salad with caramelized onions and peppers)	Total carbohydrate grams, or freebie	Sugar Calories	Points
2 cups baby spinach	freebie	0	0
Feta cheese, 2 Tbsp. crumbled	freebie	0	2
Prosciutto, 4 slices, 2 oz. diced	freebie	0	4
Parmesan cheese, 1 Tbsp.	freebie	0	0.5
Caramelized onions and red bell pepper	freebie	0	0
Meal: Dessert	Carb grams or freebie	Sugar Cals	Points
4 squares dark chocolate	5	20	1
1 glass wine, cabernet sauvignon, 5 oz.	3.6	14	3.75
Totals for day	23.6	94	34.75

APPENDIX II

FAQs and Motivation Tools

Read on for answers to my client's most common questions:

1. Can I eat as much I want of Freebies, or is there a limit?

Within reason, if a food is on the Freebies list, such as cheddar cheese, you can enjoy more than one serving. Just be aware of your body: if you feel full, stop eating.

2. What do I do if I hit a plateau?

I suggest that if you hit a plateau, return to the four-week menu to recharge your weight loss. Also, be sure to check all dressings, sauces, and drinks you are consuming for added sugars. Get back to basics and be diligent about tracking your Sugar Calories. Tracking your Sugar Calories each day will help keep you accountable and make sure that you're sticking to the 100 calorie limit. Remember, if you're near your goal weight, your weight loss will naturally slow down a bit.

Additionally, I recommend that you pay attention to how much fiber you're getting each day—aim for 25 to 30 grams to accelerate your weight loss.

3. What if I notice I'm gaining weight on this plan?

If you notice your waistline is increasing, be sure you are tracking your Sugar Calories and sticking to the 100 calorie allotment. However, it's more likely what you're measuring is actually false weight. If you add more fiber to your diet than you're used to and you aren't hydrated enough, your scale can register extra weight due to waste buildup. If you are drinking plenty of water and your elimination is still sluggish, your gut bacteria may be low (this is especially true if you've been taking antibiotics). The bacteria in your gut aid in peristalsis, which is the rhythmic contraction of the intestinal walls that literally keeps things moving. By simply adding a probiotic supplement to your diet, you can restore a healthy balance of beneficial bacteria that will make it easier for your body to clear the waste more efficiently. Also, be sure to get dietary fiber from other food sources such as vegetables like artichokes and broccoli.

4. Should I be worried about my cholesterol levels increasing on this program?

If you have high cholesterol, I recommend speaking with your doctor before starting any weight loss plan. However, it's more likely The 100™ will lower your cholesterol level rather than raise it. In fact, some studies find that highly refined carbohydrates and sugars are the largest contributors to high cholesterol. Many sugars travel directly to your liver and get converted to fat, which is sent into your blood, increasing your LDL levels (otherwise known as bad cholesterol).

5. Why do I count the calories in fruits?

If your goal is truly to get rid of body fat, then you have to limit fruits because they have sugars in them—even though these are natural sugars they can still spike your insulin levels if you eat too many of them per day. Fructose, the sugar found in fruit, has specifically been linked to increased levels of fat; since it goes directly to the liver to be processed, it gets converted to fat, which leads to excess fat and high cholesterol. Remember that fruit was created in tropical climates and in earlier times was available only certain times of the year—now we have access to everything, anytime, which is not how it was intended to be consumed.

When we look back at the 99.5 percent of our history as humans, we can see that our ancestors may have eaten lots of fruits when they were available, but that's just it, fruit was not always available, and it certainly wasn't the same types of fruits we see in the grocery stores today. Hunter-gatherers of yesterday only had sporadic access to fruits, usually berries, not the sorts of fruits we get from trees today. Apple, oranges, and bananas are high in fructose and are now available year-round. It's not how we were genetically designed to eat, and our bodies can't take the overload. In addition, the types of fruits bred today are made to be juicier and sweeter than wild varieties—and so they are more fattening. Keep this in mind when you are choosing fruits. It's a great idea to frequent farmer's markets to get seasonal fruits that haven't been modified and are organic. These fruits will be lower in sugar and healthier for you.

When you do enjoy fruit, try to eat local, seasonal fruit in its complete, natural form (with the skin on) whenever possible, and remember to minimize it in extremely high-sugar forms such as smoothies and juices.

6. Is fiber taken into account on The 100™?

Fiber is present in foods on The 100™. However, this program is all about keeping things simple. It's always best to consume carbohydrates from ideal sources such as vegetables in order to ensure you're getting a healthy amount of fiber. If you find that you are not getting the recommended amount of 25 to 30 grams of fiber, you may take a fiber supplement.

7. Where can I look up the calorie counts of foods?

The best resource to locate accurate calorie counts and other nutrient information not included in this book is at http://ndb.nal.usda.gov/ndb/foods/list.

However, these can be difficult to follow, so also try using CalorieKing.com, CalorieCount.com, or LiveStrong.com.

8. How long do I have to stay on this plan to see results?

Follow the menus and lose up to 18 pounds in two weeks. Most of my clients are so thrilled that they plan to eat this way indefinitely. Once you start employing The 100™ method you'll see results; plus, you'll feel revitalized, young, and ready for anything.

9. Do I have to exercise to lose fat?

No. Exercising is completely optional, and studies have shown that it can actually be counterproductive to weight loss. Research done at the University of Michigan revealed that typical forms of exercise don't burn enough calories to make a difference for weight-loss purposes. In fact, since it actually makes you hungrier, it can make eating the right amount of food each day difficult. Most of my clients do not exercise at all to lose weight. However, once they lost weight, many of them felt so good that they added exercise in and became addicted. See more on exercise in chapter 9.

10. What kinds of artificial sweeteners should I avoid?

You might think that the solution to avoiding sugars but still feeding your sweet tooth can be found in the many alternative sweeteners that are available. Unfortunately, this doesn't work out so well. The big three to avoid are: aspartame (NutraSweet and Equal, the blue packages), sucralose (Splenda, the yellow packages), and saccharin (Sweet'N Low, the pink packages). These substances are known as excitotoxins, which means that they "overexcite" neurons in the brain, causing degeneration and even death in important nerve cells. When too many nerve cells die, your nervous system begins to malfunction, and it can't communicate with other parts of your body. This can ultimately lead to nervous-system disorders such as Parkinson's disease, multiple sclerosis, and Alzheimer's disease. The other issue is that some scientists believe that even calorie-free, sugar-free sweeteners still spike insulin in your body, just from the sweet taste. This means that they encourage your body to store the food you are eating as stubborn fat, even if they don't add additional calories. Let's take a closer look at these three.

- **Aspartame** (Equal and NutraSweet, blue packages) This sweetener was discovered in the 1960s by a chemist who was working on an ulcer drug. Aspartame is found in thousands of food and drink products—specifically, diet sodas. Risks listed in scientific research include imbalances in your brain, migraines, mood disturbances, and insomnia. Aspartame has been linked to increased seizures, according to research in the journal *Environmental Health Perspectives.*

- **Sucralose** (Splenda, yellow packages) Discovered in 1976 by a grad student who had been told to "test" some compounds, but misunderstood and did a "taste" test instead. When he reported the sweetness, sucralose was born. This sweetener is found in more than 4,100 food products including candies, ice creams, and beverages. Sucralose is 600 times sweeter than sugar, but its health effects are anything but sweet. Good levels of naturally occurring gut bacteria (aids digestion, promotes healthy bowel movements) are reduced 50 percent by average consumers of sucralose, according to a Duke University study. The same study also showed weight gain in sucralose users.

- **Saccharin** (Sweet'N Low, pink packets) This is the oldest sugar substitute around. It was also discovered by a chemist in 1879 and became popular in the 1900s. In the 1970s, saccharin was linked to bladder cancer in animal studies, according to research published in *Science*. Instead of this resulting in banning the product, like cigarettes, saccharin packages were required to include labeling that warned consumers of the risk. This ban was removed in 1997 when the study was reviewed and found to be faulty. Still, scientists from many institutions including the University of Illinois and Boston University call for continued carcinogen warnings on saccharin based on "evidence" to suggest it's cancer causing.

11. Are there any safe sweeteners?

So what can you have that is sweet to eat? The freedom of The 100™ allows you to have modified amounts of real sugars, but it's still a good idea to limit these for all the reasons I've discussed throughout this book. If you are looking for a healthy alternative, my two favorites are stevia and xylitol, which can be found in health food stores and many supermarkets today. Stevia is an herb originally from South America; it is calorie-free, does not spike blood sugar or insulin, and can be used for baking. Plus, stevia is sweeter than sugar, so small amounts are sufficient. The FDA has approved stevia in food and drink products as the first herb-based sweetener to get such an approval. Xylitol is a sugar alcohol that is virtually calorie-free, and it doesn't spike blood sugar. Contrary to its name, xylitol doesn't contain alcohol; it's actually a type of carbohydrate. The reason this carbohydrate doesn't count is that your body can't digest it (most will be excreted in your urine). I do recommend that you keep xylitol to a minimum because some people find it causes gas and bloating when eaten in excess, so limit it to no more than 100 grams per day. There are actually three sugar alcohols you'll see in food products—here's the breakdown:

Xylitol A sugar alcohol extracted from the fiber of various fruits and vegetables.

Malitol A sugar alcohol that is popularly used in many baked goods, chocolates, and cookies. I have heard from some of my clients that this sugar alcohol can make them feel bloated. It's a harmless reaction, but an uncomfortable one, so you may want to adjust your intake of these foods.

Erythritol This sugar alcohol is known for causing less gastrointestinal disturbances, and is a good one to look for.

12. Why are Sugar Calories the same for different body sizes?

The 100™ is designed to make sure that your body is keeping insulin low and producing the appetite-suppressing hormone leptin—no matter what your gender, age, or size—while also ensuring that you get enough servings of complex carbs a day. If you have a larger body type and feel that you need more food, you can try eating more protein, fats, or some of the lower-sugar vegetables from the Freebie list. The goal is to follow The 100™ and eat until you're satisfied within those requirements. The Sugar Calories are at a level that is low enough for everyone to benefit.

13. What is the difference between The 100™ and Atkins?

Both The 100™ and Atkins focus on carbohydrates to limit insulin production, but the similarities stop there. Unlike Atkins (or South Beach) there are no phases to The 100™. This program is simply about making smarter choices from the beginning and sticking to it. Here are a few other major distinctions that make The 100™ a more healthful, more effective weight-loss program:

NO KETOSIS. The main goal of Atkins is to induce ketosis, which is a state the body enters when it is severely restricted of carbohydrates from all sources. Dieters following Atkins often buy strips that they urinate on to test for ketosis, but you won't ever be doing that on The 100™.

NO DANGEROUS ARTIFICIAL SWEETENERS. Atkins relies heavily on the use of artificial sweeteners like sucralose, while The 100™ eliminates this and all other unnatural and potentially harmful chemicals from your diet.

FLORA. The final critical element that the Atkins diet neglects to correct is the problem that causes most low-carb dieters to fail: constipation. Most people have damaged or missing gut flora, which are absolutely vital to digestion, but treat only the symptoms of the problem with excessive fiber. Without repairing flora, the transition to an ideal lifestyle free of grains and fiber supplements can be frustrating or downright impossible.

14. Can I still drink alcohol on this program?

Yes. You can still enjoy adult drinks in moderation. I suggest a glass of wine in the evening. However, if you find that you are not losing weight on this program, I recommend avoiding alcohol.

15. Do I have to give up the foods I love?

No way! You're just going to use the tracking system to keep those foods within your 100 Sugar Calories per day. By modifying your diet this way, you'll never feel deprived or hungry.

16. Why don't I track proteins and fats on this plan?

You won't be tracking proteins and fats because they don't directly affect the expansion of your waistline. Why? Various breakthrough studies done at Harvard University over the past decade have clearly shown that the main reason you have belly fat is because you've been eating too much of the wrong carbohydrates—sugar and processed carbohydrates—not too much fat or protein. It's that simple. You see, eating fats and proteins never significantly drives up the insulin level in your blood, which is the main way that your body likes to encourage the storage of fat—especially around your waistline. Bottom line: Proteins and fat are processed by your body differently. This is why the secret is to track only the Sugar Calories. Does this mean that you can eat a whole cow or ten sticks of butter? No. You need to use common sense. But the good news is that proteins and fats satiate your hunger fast, so it's almost impossible to overeat them.

17. Will this plan cost me a lot of money?

No. You can follow this plan simply by applying The 100™ to your everyday eating.

18. Will this plan work for my whole family?

Yes. The 100™ is a healthy lifestyle for everyone in your family. Monitoring the calories in hidden sugars is important to overall health for children, teens, adults, and seniors regardless of gender or body weight.

19. How can I share with you about the weight I've lost?

I'm always eager to hear about the success my clients have on this program. I encourage you to share your story along with before and after photos on my Facebook page: www.Facebook.com/JorgeCruiseFan.

20. Is this program safe for my kids?

Definitely! Limiting sugar in your children's diet and replacing it with smarter options will increase overall health both inside and out. Low-sugar, nutrient-rich foods are equally beneficial for your kids as they are for you. It may be difficult to change your kids' minds about sugar if they have fallen into a habit of constantly eating sugary snacks. Please do not let this discourage you from guiding them to a healthier lifestyle. I suggest you lead by example first. Then, get your kids involved by teaching them about the benefits of certain foods and letting them help you prepare snacks and meals. Your kids will be more interested in the foods they are eating if they help create the meals with you. Try to make cooking something fun you and your kids can enjoy together.

21. Can I be a vegan or vegetarian on this program?

Yes. Anyone can do this program. While I believe animals are the preferred source of protein, you can simply substitute the meats and/or cheeses I recommend for your own favorite vegan or vegetarian options.

22. Can I do The 100™ if I'm following a gluten-free diet?

Yes. Since the program is based on a simple, clean way of eating, it can easily be adapted to be gluten free. I encourage you to eat plenty of lean proteins and healthy fats.

23. What about leptin?

Leptin is a hormone produced by your fat cells that is supposed to signal the brain to burn more energy when its concentration is high—the more fat cells you have, the more leptin you have, and the more your brain is supposed to speed up your metabolism to burn it off. The problem is that in a diet containing high amounts of fructose, the brain becomes insensitive to leptin. Here's the kicker: When the brain can't sense the amount of leptin in your system, your brain tells you that you are hungry—starving, in fact. The brain tells your body to conserve energy, to store any fat it finds in your fat cells, and slows the rate at which you burn calories.

24. Does carbohydrate restriction work because people eat less protein and fats?

In a sense yes, but this logic is really backward. Fat accumulation in the fat cells of your body is caused by eating carbohydrates because they spike insulin, which then drives fat into your fat cells. When you change your diet around and focus on protein and fat, and keeping insulin low, you don't accumulate fat in your fat cells. When insulin is signaled it also tells you to eat more, which does make you hungrier, so while proteins and fats are slower to digest, and may in this sense help you to eat less, they also are foods that don't spike hunger signals or cravings in your body the way that carbohydrates do.

25. If I am thin, I don't need to worry about eating this way, right?

Not true. There are people who are genetically destined to store less food as fat, even if they eat a highly refined, easily digestible diet of carbohydrates. We've known for a long time that there is a genetic component to being fat or thin. This is often seen in teenagers, and you'll hear middle-aged people saying, "I used to be able to eat anything when I was younger." Just because you can eat junk foods without gaining weight doesn't mean you are healthy. You can still have high levels of heart clogging fats from the overconsumption of sugary foods and refined starches. This is especially concerning in teens because they think that they can just catch up and eat healthy later in life, and parents often go along with this thinking, but in reality they are laying the foundation for insulin resistance and glucose intolerance, which will make them more likely to struggle with obesity, diabetes, heart disease, cancer, and so on in the later years of their life. It's just that their bodies are growing, so fuel is being partitioned differently than it will be when they get older. So, thin or fat, we all need to reduce our intake of fattening carbohydrates to protect our health.

APPENDIX III

Resources

The Belly Fat Cure™: Discover the New Carb Swap System and Lose 4 to 9 Lbs. Every Week by Jorge Cruise (2009). Learn how you are eating foods packed with hidden sweeteners that cause weight gain, and easy ways to get rid of them. This simple guide gives effortless and affordable smart eating tips. It includes more than 1,100 options menus for carboholics, meat lovers, chicken and seafood fans, chocoholics, fast-food junkies, and even vegans.

The Belly Fat Cure™ Quick Meals: Lose 4 to 9 Lbs. a Week with On-the-Go CARB SWAPS by Jorge Cruise (2011). Based on *The Belly Fat Cure*, this book gives you options to eat on-the-go with hundreds of meals from popular chains and restaurants, as well as convenience meals you can find in your supermarket.

The Belly Fat Cure™ Fast Track: Discover the Ultimate Carb Swap and Drop Up to 14 Lbs. the First 14 Days by Jorge Cruise (2011). This doctor-approved, science-based solution includes yummy foods such as cookies, pancakes, burgers, and even wine. This book includes an extensive guide for super fast foods you already have in your kitchen.

The Belly Fat Cure™ Sugar & Carb Counter: Discover Which Foods Will Melt Up to 9 Lbs. This Week by Jorge Cruise (2010). A fantastic resource guide, this book contains hundreds of products from your supermarket, menu items from restaurants, coffee bars, and fast food chains that show their sugar and carb counts.

Practical Paleo: A Customized Approach to Health and a Whole-Foods Lifestyle by Diane Sanfilippo, Bill Staley, and Robb Wolf (2012). This book explains why avoiding both processed foods and foods marketed as healthy—like grains, legumes, and pasteurized dairy—will improve how you look and feel and lead to lasting weight loss. Practical Paleo is jam-packed with over 120 easy recipes, all with special notes about common food allergens. Meal plans are also included.

Paleo Comfort Foods: Homestyle Cooking for a Gluten-Free Kitchen by Julie Sullivan Mayfield, Charles Mayfield, Mark Adams, and Robb Wolf (2011). An arsenal of recipes that are healthy crowd-pleasers, and appeal to those following a Paleo, primal, or gluten-free way of life. This book implements Paleo guidelines and principles (no grains, no gluten, no legumes, and no dairy). The Mayfields give you 100+ recipes and full-color photos with entertaining stories throughout.

Why We Get Fat: And What to Do About It by Gary Taubes (2011). Building upon his critical work in *Good Calories, Bad Calories* and presenting fresh evidence for his claim, Gary Taubes revisits the question of what's making us fat—and how we can change. He reveals the bad nutritional science of the last century—none more damaging or misguided than the "calories-in, calories-out" model of why we get fat—and the good science that has been ignored.

Good Calories, Bad Calories: Fats, Carbs, and the Controversial Science of Diet and Health by Gary Taubes (2008). In this book, Taubes argues that the problem with obesity lies in refined carbohydrates, like white flour, easily digested starches, and sugars, and that the key to good health is in the kind of calories we take in, not the number of calories we consume or burn off through exercise.

Sweet and Dangerous by John Yudkin (1978). When this book was first published, it was hugely controversial because it put sugar on the witness stand the way no other book had ever done before. The back cover has this to say: "Dr. John Yudkin, a renowned physician, biochemist, and researcher whose pioneering studies in sugar have been recognized throughout the world, offers never-before-published findings about sugar and explains, clearly and concisely, why ordinary table sugar is a critical health issues for all ages."

Primal Body, Primal Mind: Beyond the Paleo Diet for Total Health and a Longer Life by Nora T. Gedgaudas (2011). This book provides sustainable diet strategies to curb sugar cravings, promote fat burning and weight loss, reduce stress and anxiety, improve sleep and moods, increase energy and immunity, and enhance memory and brain function. In addition, Gedgaudas discusses how our modern diet leads to weight gain and diseases of civilization. She also examines the healthy lives of our pre-agricultural Paleolithic ancestors and the marked decline in stature, bone density, and dental health and the increase in birth defects, malnutrition, and disease following the implementation of the agricultural lifestyle.

Sugar Blues by William F. Duffy (1986). A book that was inspired by the crusade of Hollywood legend Gloria Swanson. It is a classic exposé that argues that sugar is our generation's greatest medical killer and shows how a revitalizing, sugar-free diet can not only change lives, but quite possibly save them.

In Defense of Food: An Eater's Manifesto by Michael Pollan (2009). In his book, Pollan proposes an answer to the question of what we should eat. Pollan's manifesto shows us how we can start making thoughtful food choices that will enrich our lives, enlarge our sense of what it means to be healthy, and bring pleasure back to eating.

The Omnivore's Dilemma: A Natural History of Four Meals by Michael Pollan (2007). In this book, Pollan asks the question, what we should have for dinner? To learn the answer, Pollan follows each of the food chains that sustain us throughout their origins to the dinner plate—industrial food, organic food, and food we forage ourselves—and, in the process, writes a critique of the American way of eating.

Food Rules: An Eater's Manual by Michael Pollan (2009). This book offers 64 rules on eating based on Pollan's previous book, *In Defense of Food*. There are three sections: eat food, mostly plants, not too much. The book also discusses the "diseases of affluence" to the diet of processed meats and food products, and offers its rules as a remedy to the problem.

Ending the Food Fight: Guide Your Child to a Healthy Weight in a Fast Food/ Fake Food World by David Ludwig and Suzanne Rostler (2008). Dr. David Ludwig's lifestyle plan for eating has benefited thousands of families. Here Ludwig shares a 9-week program, including recipes, motivational tips, and activities that help families eat healthier.

The Diet Myth by Paul Campos (2004), an exposé on the hysteria surrounding weight and health in the Western world today. Includes reviews of medical studies and interviews with leading doctors, scientists, eating-disorder specialists, and psychiatrists on dieting, weight loss, and obesity.

Mindless Eating: Why We Eat More Than We Think by Brian Wansink (2006). In his book, food psychologist Brian Wansink shows why you may not realize how much you're eating, what you're eating, or why you're even eating at all.

Eat Stop Eat by Brad Pilon (2012). This ebook reviews research on the benefits of intermittent fasting, includes a detailed program for including two 24-hour fasting days per week.

Websites

www.jorgecruise.com Please use my website for many resources including recipes, interviews with experts, and sign up to join my free club and get tips and helpful coaching.

http://michaelpollan.com See more from the author of *Food Rules: An Eater's Manual* (2010). On his website, you can find many links to articles, resources and locations where he is speaking.

www.garytaubes.com Follow the author of *Good Calorie, Bad Calorie* and *Why We Got Fat* as he updates you on the latest happenings in health. Gary's website includes lectures, articles, and ongoing blogs.

http://youtube/dBnniua6-oM Robert Lustig's viral video on YouTube: "Sugar: The Bitter Truth."

www.eatwellguide.org/i.php?pd=Home A directory of sustainably raised meat, poultry, dairy, and eggs.

www.eatwild.com A source for safe, healthy, natural, and nutritious grass-fed beef, lamb, goats, bison, poultry, pork, dairy, and other wild edibles.

APPENDIX IV

Glossary

Adipose Tissue Body fat or fat cells. Composed of 80 percent, this is the storage site for triglycerides and fatty acids. Its main role is to store and provide energy in the form of fats (lipids), although it also cushions organs and insulates the body.

Adipocytes Fat cells, body fat, or lipocytes (see above).

Amino Acids The building blocks of all protein. There are 9 essential amino acids that the body cannot make itself and that must be provided by the food we eat.

Antioxidants Antioxidants are substances that may protect cells from the damage caused by unstable molecules known as free radicals. Examples include beta-carotene, lycopene, vitamins C, E, and A.

Arteriosclerosis The thickening and hardening of arteries caused by plaques on the inner lining of major blood vessels.

Atherosclerosis A disease of the arteries characterized by plaques of fatty material on their inner walls.

Blood pressure The pressure of the blood within the arteries. It is produced primarily by the contraction of the heart muscle, and measured by two numbers. The first (systolic pressure) is measured after the heart contracts and is highest. The second (diastolic pressure) is measured before the heart contracts and is lowest. A blood pressure cuff is used to measure the pressure. Elevation of blood pressure is called hypertension.

Body mass index (BMI) A key for relating weight to height. BMI is a person's weight in kilograms (kg) divided by his or her height in meters squared. The National Institutes of Health (NIH) now defines normal weight, overweight, and obesity according to BMI rather than the traditional height/weight charts. Overweight is a BMI of 27.3 or more for women and 27.8 or more for men. Obesity is a BMI of 30 or more for either sex (about 30 pounds overweight).

Calorie A unit of measurement. Typical defined as the unit of heat energy required to raise 1 kilogram of water 1 degree Celsius.

Carbohydrates Compounds of carbon, hydrogen, and oxygen that make up sugars, starches, plants, and fruits.

Cholesterol A waxy substance produced by the liver and found in the blood.

The Cochrane Collaboration An international network of more than 28,000 experts from over 100 countries. The collaboration publishes objective scientific reviews to help provide well-informed advice about health care. You can find reviews online in the *Cochrane Database of Systematic Reviews*, at www .cochrane.org/cochrane-reviews/about-cochrane-library. This organization is one of the most respected for its unbiased objective scientific reviews in the world.

Complex carbohydrate A carbohydrate that has a more complex structure to include fiber, starch, or glycogen. These complex carbs still increase the production of insulin.

Diabetes, Type I A disease characterized by the lack of insulin and resulting in elevated blood glucose levels.

Diabetes, Type II A disease characterized by resistance of the cells in the body to insulin; type 2 diabetes also leads to elevated blood sugar levels.

Endocrine glands A special group of cells that make hormones. The major endocrine glands are the pituitary, pineal, thymus, thyroid, adrenal, and pancreas. In addition, men produce hormones in their testes and women produce them in their ovaries.

The endocrine system The system that controls all the chemical messengers that tells your body what to do (via hormones). The endocrine system has four functions: 1) controls reproduction, 2) regulates growth and development of all cells, 3) maintains the internal environment (temperature, hydration), and 4) regulates energy production, utilization, and storage.

Energy The power that we obtain from food and convert into movement, functions, and thoughts.

Energy deficit The state of having expended more energy than you've consumed. Energy deficit results in hunger, or conservation of energy (sedentary behavior).

False belly fat Trapped waste matter that adds pounds and inches to the belly, and can also interfere with the absorption of nutrients and a healthy digestion.

Free fatty acids Fat that is freely flowing in the blood on its way to becoming storage, or being used for fuel.

Fructose A simple sugar found in fruits, table sugar, and high-fructose corn syrup. Fructose doesn't spike insulin the same way glucose does. See page 61 for more information.

Glucagon The body's mechanism for shrinking fat tissue. This hormone is secreted by the pancreas and helps regulate blood sugar and metabolizes stored fat, but it is only capable of unlocking energy from fat cells when insulin levels are low.

Glucose The form in which sugar circulates in the bloodstream—this is the body's first energy source.

Glycemic index An index designed to identify how rapidly a food is digested into glucose, and how much it causes blood sugar to rise.

Glyceride A group name for fats including monoglycerides, diglycerides, and triglycerides. These contain two or three fatty acids.

Glycerol-3-phospate A metabolic product that occurs when glucose transforms into triglycerides.

Glycogen A complex form of glucose that is stored in the liver and muscles to be used as fuel to meet energy needs.

High-density lipoprotein (HDL) Lipoproteins (a combination of fat and protein) that carry cholesterol from the cells to the liver for breakdown and elimination from the body. Thought to protect against heart disease.

Hormone Hormones are chemical messengers that travel in your bloodstream to tissues or organs and tell your body what it needs to do regarding growth and development, metabolism (how your body gets energy from the foods you eat), sexual function, reproduction, and mood.

Hormone-sensitive lipase (HSL) An enzyme that works to make fat cells leaner. This molecule lives inside fat cells, and its job is to break down triglycerides (bulky fats inside fat tissue and the liver). It is inhibited by the presence of insulin (hence the name, it is "sensitive" to insulin).

Homeostasis This is how a cell regulates its internal conditions to maintain a state of healthy equilibrium or stability despite outside external changing conditions. This usually works through a system of feedback controls—in the human body: the endocrine system, nervous system, digestive system, circulatory system, and so on. A good example is the way the body regulates temperature in an effort to maintain around 98.6°F. We sweat to cool off during the hot summer days, and we shiver to produce heat during the cold winter season (and that is homeostasis in action).

Hyperglycemia Abnormally elevated glucose (blood sugar).

Hyperinsulinemia Chronically high levels of insulin in the body.

Hyperlipidemia Abnormally elevated blood fats, most often either low-density lipoproteins or triglycerides.

Hypoglycemia A chronically low level of blood glucose (blood sugar) in the body.

Hypothalamus This almond-size section of the brain is the control center for numerous critical functions in the body. It communicates with the nervous system, the endocrine system, and all the other systems in the body to maintain a state of healthy equilibrium (homeostasis). This area of the brain communicates through hormones and nerve impulses with other areas of your body to regulate body temperature, hunger, moods, sex drive, sleep, and thirst.

Insulin The regulator of blood sugar, this hormone, which is secreted by the pancreas, also drives cells to burn carbohydrates instead of fat, and indirectly stimulates the production of more fat. The chronic elevation of this hormone (caused by consuming carbohydrates) sets off a chain reaction that negatively impacts almost every part of the body.

Insulin resistance The failure of insulin to exert its normal effect on cells. This causes a rise in blood sugar levels and therefore triggers the pancreas to release more insulin.

Intermittent fasting The act of abstaining from food, and all caloric beverages, for 24 to 36 hours, usually the former, once or twice per week. Results in increased insulin sensitivity, lower blood sugar, increased weight loss, and reduced disease, without decreasing metabolism.

Ketone bodies Three chemicals that are produced as by-products when fatty acids are broken down for energy. These are soluble compounds, and their production is referred to as ketogenesis. When excess ketone bodies accumulate, this abnormal (but not necessarily harmful) state is called ketosis. When even larger amounts of ketone bodies accumulate, it is called ketoacidosis.

Ketoacidosis A state of extremely high ketone bodies. High levels of ketones cause the blood to become more acidic. This is also referred to as diabetic ketoacidosis, or DKA, when uncontrolled diabetes is the cause. Ketoacidosis is a severe life-threatening condition requiring immediate treatment. Symptoms of ketoacidosis include nausea, vomiting, abdominal pain, rapid breathing, and, in severe cases, unconsciousness.

Ketosis A state the body enters when it is severely restricted of carbohydrates from all sources.

Lipase An enzyme secreted by the pancreas that aids the digestion of fats.

Lipid A fat of either plant or animal origin.

Lipogenesis The formation of fat from glucose.

Lipolysis The breakdown of triglycerides to free fatty acids and glycerol, both of which are used as fuel in the body.

Lipoproteins A combination of fat and proteins in the body that circulates in the bloodstream. Lipoproteins are the primary carriers of lipids.

Lipoprotein lipase (LPL) An enzyme that aids in the storage of fat. LPLs lives on the exterior of liver, fat, and muscle cells. They are stimulated by insulin to bring in fuel to be stored as fat.

Low-density lipoproteins (LDL) Lipoproteins are important in the transport of cholesterol. There are two different types of LDLs, large fluffy types that don't seem to play a role in heart disease, and small dense LDLs (see very low-density lipoproteins) that do.

Low-carb diet A broad term that encompasses many diets that focus on reducing both simple and complex carbohydrates in order to lose weight.

Maltose The fundamental structural unit of glycogen and starch, it is made of two molecules of glucose.

Metabolic syndrome Also called Syndrome X. A collection of the following: insulin resistance, elevated insulin levels (hyperinsulinemia), elevated triglycerides, obesity, and glucose resistance.

Metabolism The sum of all the chemical and physiological processes by which the body grows and maintains itself, and the processes and energy used to break matter down into a new state.

Minerals There are two kinds of minerals: macrominerals and trace minerals. Macrominerals are the minerals your body requires in larger amounts, and there are many types including calcium, phosphorus, magnesium, sodium, potassium, chloride and sulfur. Trace minerals are needed by your body in smaller amounts, and these include iron, manganese, copper, iodine, zinc, cobalt, fluoride, and selenium. Your body uses minerals to help with many purposes such as building bones, making hormones, and regulating your heartbeat.

Monounsaturated fats Fat molecules containing only one double bond. For example, olive oil, peanuts, and walnuts.

Opioids Any external substance that numbs pain and creates a feeling of euphoria, typically by mimicking the body's endorphins—opioids stimulate the reward center of the brain. Some scientists believe that sugar and fructose act as opioids in the brain.

Paleolithic diet A diet based on the nutrition available to the human species more than 10,000 years ago, before the birth of farming. This diet restricts foods that only became available due to modern agricultural and industrial processes.

Pancreas An important organ that produces both insulin and glucagon, as well as digestive enzymes such as lipase (an enzyme that helps digest fats).

Phosphatidylinositol 3-kinases An enzyme called PI3 kinase for short that regulates a cell's sensitivity to insulin, and also turns out to be a cancer-promoting gene.

Plaque Deposits of cholesterol, calcium, and blood clot on the lining of major vessels, also called atheroma.

Saturated fats Fat molecules containing carbon atoms that are fully bound with hydrogen atoms, found in most animal fats.

Simple carbohydrates Most commonly referred to as sugar and quickly absorbed into the bloodstream. These refined, easily digestible starches and sugars spike insulin to unhealthy levels.

Simple sugars Also called monosaccharides. Glucose, fructose, and galactose (milk sugar) are the main sugars.

Smart Sugar Calories These are from the best sources of counted Sugar Calories. Including beans and legumes, starchy vegetables, fruit and whole grains. When choosing to have Sugar Calories these are the most nutritious sources of counted foods. Try choosing these instead of ice cream and cake when possible.

Syndrome X Also called metabolic syndrome. A collection of the following: insulin resistance, elevated insulin levels (hyperinsulinemia), elevated triglycerides, obesity, and glucose resistance.

Synthesis The manufacture or creation of a new substance.

Trans fats Fats similar to saturated fats, produced by heating oil. Trans fats increase LDL and reduce HDL.

Triglycerides A bulky fat that is stored in the fat cells and made by the liver, comprised of three fatty acids and a bond of glycerol.

Very low-density lipoproteins (VLDL) Heart harming lipoproteins that are involved in the transportation of fatty components from the liver to fat cells.

BIBLIOGRAPHY

Abbott, Elizabeth. 2009. *Sugar: A Bittersweet History*. London and New York: Duckworth Overlook.

Adas, Michael, ed. 2001. *Agricultural and Pastoral Societies in Ancient and Classical History*. Philadelphia: Temple University Press.

Agriculture Fact Book. 2001–2002. March 2003. Washington, DC: United States Department of Agriculture, Office of Communications. Chapter 2. Retrieved from www.usda.gov/factbook/2002factbook.pdf.

Albert R. Mann Library. 2012. Core Historical Literature of Agriculture (CHLA). Ithaca, NY: Albert R. Mann Library, Cornell University. http://chla.library.cornell.edu (version January 2005).

Anson, M. R. 2003. "Intermittent fasting dissociates beneficial effects of dietary restriction on glucose metabolism and neuronal resistance to injury from calorie intake." *Proceedings of the National Academy of Sciences of the United States of America*. 100(10): 6216–6220.

Anson, R. S. 1972. *McGovern: A Biography*. New York: Holt, Rinehart and Winston, pp. 218–242.

Aubrey, A. 2006, November 16. "Teaching Kids the Science of Calories." *National Public Radio*. Retrieved from www.npr.org/templates/story/story.php?storyId=6493713.

Avena, N. M., Rava, P., and Hoebel, B. G. 2008. "Evidence for sugar addiction: Behavioral and neurochemical effects of intermittent, excessive sugar intake." *Neuroscience and Biobehavioral Reviews*. 32(1):20–39.

Banting, W. 1869. *Letter on Corpulence, Addressed to the Public*. 4th edition. London: Harrison. Republished New York: 2005. Retrieved from www.lowcarb.ca/corpulence/index.html.

Barnes, A. C. 1974. *The Sugar Cane*. London: Leonard Hill Books.

Bernard, C. 1974. *Phenomena of Life Common to Animals and Vegetables.* Translated by R. P. Cook, and M. A. Cook, Dundee: R. P. and M. A. Cook. [Originally published in 1878.]

Beulens, J. W. J., et al. 2007. "High dietary glycemic load and glycemic index increase risk of cardiovascular disease among middle-aged women." *Journal of the American College of Cardiology.* 50(1):14–21.

Bichsel, S. E. 1988. "An overview of the U.S. beet sugar industry." *Chemistry and Processing of Sugarbeet and Sugarcane,* ed. M. A. Clarke and M. A. Godshall, 1–7. Amsterdam: Elsevier.

Brehm, B. J., et al. 2003. "A randomized trial comparing a very low carbohydrate diet and a calorie-restricted low fat diet on body weight and cardiovascular risk factors in healthy women." *Journal of Clinical Endocrinology & Metabolism.* 88(4):1617–1623.

Brillat-Savarin, J. A. 1986. *The Physiology of Taste.* Translated by M. F. K. Fisher. San Francisco: North Point Press. [Originally published in 1825.]

Cahill, G. F., et al. 1959, September 25. "Effects of insulin on adipose tissue." *Annals of the New York Academy of Sciences.* 82:4303–4311.

Centers for Disease Control and Prevention. 2012, December 11. *Carbohydrates.* Retrieved from Nutrition for Everyone at www.cdc.gov/nutrition/everyone/basics/carbs.html.

Cloud, J. 2009, August 9. "Why exercise won't make you thin." *Time Magazine.* Retrieved from www.time.com/time/printout/0,8816,1914974,00.html.

Cohn, V. 1980, August 31. "A passion to keep fit: 100 million Americans exercising." *Washington Post.*

Cordain, L, et al. 2000. "Plant-animal subsistence ratios and macronutrient energy estimations in worldwide hunter-gatherer diets." *American Journal of Clinical Nutrition.* 71(3):682–692.

Dancel, J. F. 1864. *Obesity, or Excessive Corpulence: The Various Causes and the Rational Means of Cure.* Translated by Barrett, M. Toronto: W. C. Chewett.

Diamond, D. 2011, May 20. "How Bad Science and Big Business Created the Obesity Epidemic." University of South Florida, College of Arts and Sciences. Retrieved from www.youtube.com/watch?v=3vr-c8GeT34.

Dietler, Michael, and Brian Hayden, eds. *Feasts*: *Archaeological and Ethno-*

graphic Perspectives on Food, Politics, and Power. Washington, DC: Smithsonian Institution Press, 2001.

Donaldson, B. F. 1962. *Strong Medicine.* Garden City, NY: Doubleday

Ebbeling, C. B., et al. 2012. Effects of dietary composition on energy expenditure during weight-loss maintenance. *Journal of the American Medical Association.* 307(24):2627–2634.

Fogelholm, M. & Kukkonen-Harjula, K. 2000. "Does physical activity prevent weight gain—a systematic review." *Obesity Reviews.* 1(2):95–111.

Greene, R. 1951. *The Practice of Endocrinology.* Philadelphia: Lippincott.

Haist, R. E. & Best, C. H. 1966. Carbohydrate Metabolism and Insulin. *The Physiological Basis of Medical Practice,* 8th edition, Best, C. H. & Taylor, N. M., eds. Baltimore: Williams & Wilkins.

Hargrove, J. L. 2006. "History of the calorie in nutrition." *Journal of Nutrition.* 136:2957–2961.

Harvard School of Public Health. 2013. The Nutrition Source. *Carbohydrates: Good Carbs Guide the Way.* Retrieved from www.hsph.harvard.edu/nutritionsource/carbohydrates-full-story/.

Harvey, W. 1872. *On Corpulence in Relation to Disease: With Some Remarks on Diet.* London: Henry Renshaw.

Harvie, M. N., et al. 2011. "The effects of intermittent or continuous energy restriction on weight loss and metabolic disease risk markers: a randomized trial in young overweight women." *International Journal of Obesity.* 35(5):714–727.

Hayden, Brian. "The cultural capacities of neandertals: a review and re-evaluation." *Journal of Human Evolution.* 24(1993):11346.

Hazen, T. R. 1999. The History of Flour Milling In Early America. Retrieved from www.angelfire.com/journal/millrestoration/history.html.

Higginson, J. 1997. "From geographical pathology to environmental carcinogenesis: a historical reminiscence. *Cancer Letters.* 117:133–42.

Hoffman, F. L. 1937. *Cancer and Diet.* Baltimore: Williams & Wilkins.

Howard, J. M. 2012. *The History of the Pancreas.* The Pancreas Club: Los Angeles, CA. Retrieved from http://pancreasclub.com/home/pancreas/.

Indiana University. 2010, August 24. "Obesity, Type 2 Diabetes, and Fructose." Office of Science Outreach; Dept. of Biology. The Trustees of Indiana University. Retrieved from www.indiana.edu/~oso/Fructose/Consequences.html.

Johnson, R. K., et al. 2009. Dietary Sugars Intake and Cardiovascular Health: A Scientific Statement From the American Heart Association. *Circulation.* Retrieved from http://circ.ahajournals.org/content/120/11/1011.full.pdf. DOI: 10.1161/CIRCULATIONAHA.109.192627.

Kennedy, E. T., et al. 2001, April. "Popular diets: correlation to health, nutrition, and obesity." *Journal of the American Dietetic Association.* 101(4):411–420.

Keys, A. 1980. *Seven Countries: A Multivariate Analysis of Death and Coronary Heart Disease.* Cambridge, MA: Harvard University Press.

Keys, A., et al. 1950. *The Biology of Human Starvation*, Vols. I–II. Minneapolis, MN: University of Minnesota Press.

Kipple, K. F. and Ornelas, K. C., 2000, December. *The Cambridge World History of Food.* New York, NY: Cambridge University Press. www.cambridge .org/us/books/kiple/sugar.htm.

Larsson, S. C., Bergkvist, L., and Wolk, A. 2006. "Consumption of sugar and sugar-sweetened foods and the risk of pancreatic cancer in a prospective study." *American Journal of Clinical Nutrition.* 84(5):1171–1176.

Leibel, R. L., Rosenbaum, M., and Hirsch, J. 1995. "Changes in energy expenditure resulting from altered body weight." *New England Journal of Medicine.* 332(10):621–628.

Levi, B. and Werman, M. J. 1998. "Long-term fructose consumption accelerates glycation and several age-related variables in male rats." *Journal of Nutrition.* 128:1442–1449.

Lewis, G. F., et al. 2002. "Disordered fat storage and mobilization in the pathogenesis of insulin resistance and type 2 diabetes." *Endocrine Reviews.* 23(2):201–209. Retrieved from http://edrv.endojournals.org/content/23/2/201 .full.pdf+html.

Malik, V. S. and Hu, F. B. 2012. "Sweeteners and risk of obesity and type 2 diabetes: the role of sugar-sweetened beverages." *Current Diabetes Reports.* 12(2):195–203.

Maratos-Flier, E. and Flier, J. S. 2005. Obesity. *Joslin's Diabetes Mellitus.* 533–545.

Martin, A., et al. 2000. "Is advice for breakfast consumption justified? Results from a short-term dietary and metabolic experiment in young healthy men." *British Journal of Nutrition*. 84(3):337–344

McCall, N., ed. 1993. *The Portrait Collection of Johns Hopkins Medicine: A Catalog of Paintings and Photographs at The Johns Hopkins University School of Medicine and The Johns Hopkins Hospital*. Baltimore: The Johns Hopkins University School of Medicine.

Moyer, M. W. 2010, May. "Carbs against cardio: more evidence that refined carbohydrates, not fats, threaten the heart." *Scientific American*. Retrieved from www.scientificamerican.com/article.cfm?id=carbs-against-cardio.

National Institutes of Health: The U.S. National Library of Medicine. 2012, May 16. *Carbohydrates*. Retrieved from Medline Plus at www.nlm.nih .gov/medlineplus/ency/article/002469.htm.

Newburgh, L. H. 1948. "Energy metabolism in obese patients." *Bulletin of the New York Academy of Medicine*. 24(4):227–38.

———. 1930. "The nature of obesity." *Journal of Clinical Investigation*. 8(2):197–213. doi:10.1172/JCI100260.

Nobel Lectures. 1965. "Frederick G. Banting—Biography." *Physiology or Medicine 1922–1941*. Amsterdam: Elsevier Publishing Company. Retrieved from www.nobelprize.org/nobel_prizes/medicine/laureates/1923/banting-bio .html.

O'Connell, J. and Hawkes, K. 1981. "Alyawara plant use and optimal foraging theory." In *Hunter-Gatherer Foraging Strategies*. Edited by Bruce Winterhalder and Eric Smith. Chicago: University of Chicago Press.

Osler, W. 1901. *The Principles and Practice of Medicine*. New York: D. Appleton.

Oz, M. 2011, February 24. Gary Taubes on *The Dr. Oz Radio Show*. Why We Get Fat, Part 1. Retrieved from www.youtube.com/watch?feature=endscre en&v=lMUGUZ3EEEo&NR=1.

Pennington, A. W. 1953. "Treatment of obesity with calorie unrestricted diets." *American Journal of Clinical Nutrition*. 1(5):343–348.

Pirozzo, S., et al. 2002. Advice on low-fat diets for obesity. *Cochrane Database System Review*. (2):CD003640. DOI:10.1002/14651858.

Ponting, Clive. 2000. *World History: A New Perspective*. London: Chatto & Windus.

Reaven G. M. 1988. Banting lecture 1988. Role of insulin resistance in human disease. *Diabetes* 37:1595–607.

Rose, G. 1985. "Sick individuals and sick populations." *International Journal of Epidemiology*. International Epidemiological Association. 14(1).

Rosenbloom, S. 2010, March 23. "Calorie data to be posted at most chains." *New York Times*. Retrieved from www.nytimes.com/2010/03/24/business/24menu.html?_r=0.

Russell, F. 1975. *The Pima Indians*. Tucson: University of Arizona Press. [Originally published 1908.]

Samaha, F. F., et al. 2003, May 22. "A low-carbohydrate as compared with a low-fat diet in severe obesity." *New England Journal of Medicine*. 348:2074–2081.

Sanchez, A., et al. 1973. "Role of sugars in human neutrophilic phagocytosis." *American Journal of Clinical Nutrition*. 26(11): 180–1184.

Schernhammer, E.S., et al. 2005. "Sugar-sweetened soft drink consumption and risk of pancreatic cancer in two prospective cohorts." *Cancer Epidemiology, Biomarkers, & Prevention*. 14(9):2098–2105.

Schulze M. B., et al. 2004, August 25. "Sugar-sweetened beverages, weight gain, and incidence of type 2 diabetes in young and middle-aged women." *Journal of the American Medical Association*. 292(8):927–34.

Strom, S. 2012, September 12. "McDonald's menu to post calorie data." *New York Times*. Retrieved from www.nytimes.com/2012/09/13/business/mcdonalds-to-start-posting-calorie-counts.html.

Tanner, T. 1869. *The Practice of Medicine*. Oxford University Press: Henry Renshaw. Retrieved from http://books.google.com/books?id=5RsDAAAAQAAJ&oe=UTF-8.

Tappy, L. and Jéquier, E. 1993, November. "Fructose and dietary thermogenesis." *American Journal of Clinical Nutrition*. 58(5 supplement):766s–770s.

Taubes, G. 2007. *Good Calories, Bad Calories: Fats, Carbs, and the Controversial Science of Diet and Health*. New York: Anchor Books.

———. 2011, February 17. "Is sugar toxic?" *New York Times*. Retrieved from www.nytimes.com/2011/04/17/magazine/mag-17Sugar-t.html?_r=0#.

————. 2011. *Why We Get Fat: And What to Do About It.* New York: Anchor Books.

Trapp, E. G., et al. 2008. "The effects of high-intensity intermittent exercise training on fat loss and fasting insulin levels of young women." *International Journal of Obesity.* 32(4):684–691.

Sharpe, P. 1998. *Sugar Cane: Past and Present.* Illinois: Southern Illinois University.

Speth, J. and Spielmann, K. 1983. "Energy source, protein metabolism, and hunter-gatherer subsistence strategies." *Journal of Anthropological Archaeology* 2.

U.S. Senate Select Committee on Nutrition and Human Needs. 1977. *Dietary Goals for the United States. 2nd edition.* Washington (DC): U.S. Government Printing Office.

Verboeket-van de, W. P. and Westerterp, K. R. 1993. "Frequency of feeding, weight reduction and energy metabolism." *International Journal of Obesity and Related Metabolic Disorders.* 17(1):31–36.

Williams, W. R. 1908. *The Natural History of Cancer with Special Reference to Its Causation and Prevention.* London: William Heinemann.

Young, C. M., Ringler, I., Greer, B. J. 1953. "Reducing and post-reducing maintenance on the moderate fat diet: metabolic studies." *Journal of the American Dietetic Association.* 29(9):890–96.

ACKNOWLEDGMENTS

A huge, heartfelt thank you to the wonderful HarperCollins team: Amy Bendell, Paige Hazzan, Mary Schuck, Lorie Young, Jamie Kerner, Nyamekye Waliyaya, Liate Stehlik, Lynn Grady, Judy DeGrottole, Shelby Meizlik, and most especially to my dear friend, Lisa Sharkey, the world's best editor, who was a true visionary for The 100™. Thanks to your belief in this project and your work to shift the misperception of calories, I know we can change health and well-being on a global level; I can't thank you enough for your support and your passion.

I owe particular gratitude to my amazing team, whom without, nothing would be possible. To Kristin Penne, for keeping us all organized, on time, and sane. Your support and assistance means so much. To Oliver Stephenson, for your direction, support, and assistance, I couldn't do it without you. You truly know how to apply your incredible commitment and talent to our mission. You make it all run! And to Marianne McGinnis, without your hard work and dedication, this book would not exist. Your attention to detail and incredible research were invaluable and you have made this book what it is. You are my core team, and your hard work and incredible talent were irreplaceable to this project; I can't thank you all enough for your dedication and commitment to creating outstanding content.

A very special thank you to my invaluable circle of experts: Gary Taubes, Dr. Robert Lustig, Dr. Mehmet Oz, Dr. Nicholas Perricone, Dr. Christiane Northrup, Dr. David Ludwig, and Michael Pollan. Thank you to Dr. Vincent Pedre for your incredible insight, feedback, and the beautiful foreword. It means so much. And to Dr. Andrew Weil, thank you for your constant support and feedback.

To my clients—your support in helping me refine this program, offering your comments, tips, and the courage to change your own lives have been a gift—thank you. You all inspire me each and every day.

I wish to thank so many others who have contributed to this book as well as my overall vision and mission. Their advice, knowledge, and support have been so valuable and I would not be where I am today without them. While the list could go on and on, I wish to thank a few of them here, in alphabetical order.

Abra Potkin

Al Roker

Alexandra Cohen

Allison Markowitz

Andy Jenkins

Anthony Robbins

Bill Geddie

Blair Atkins

Bob Wietrak

Bobbi Brown

Bobby Flay

Bruce Barlean

Carol Brooks

Cathy Chermol

Chef Art Smith

Chef Emeril Lagasse

Chris Hendrickson

Chris Park

Clate Mask

Daniel Sheldon

David Tompson

Diane Sawyer

Dustin Nigilo

Eben Pagan

Evan Dollard

Frank Kern

Ginnie Roeglin

Hanna Richert

Heather Spangler

Hillary Estey McLoughlin

Howard Bragman

Jacqui Stafford

Jaireck Robbins

Janet Annino

Jared Davis

Jay Robb

Joanna Parides

Joe Fusco

John Redmann

Jon Davidson

Jose Pretlow

Joseph Pappa

Joseph Quesada

Katie Couric

Kelly Ripa

Kenny Rueter

Kirk Masters

Lance Bass & the Dirty Pop
    Team @ Sirius Satellite
    Radio

Leslie Marcus

Linda Fennell

Lisa Gregorisch-Dempsey

Louise Hay

Maggie Jaqua

Marc Victor

Mario Batali

Mark Sisson

Marta Fox

Martha Stewart

Mary-Ellen Keating

Maura Wogan

Mel Maurer

Michael Koenings

Michelle McGowen

Natalie Morales

Oprah Winfrey

Pennie Ianniciello

President Bill Clinton

Preston Stapley

Rachael Ray

Richard Galanti

Richard Heller

Robbie McMillin

Robin Mead

Robin Roberts

Sage Robbins

Scott Eason

Scott Martineau

Stephen Steigler

Suzanne Somers

Suze Orman

Terence Noonan

Tim Austgen

Tim Mantoani

Tom Blair

Toni Richi

Travis Rosser

Wayne Dyer

FOLLOW JORGE AT

Facebook.com/JorgeCruiseFan

ABOUT THE AUTHOR

JORGE CRUISE is the #1 *New York Times* bestselling author of more than fifteen weight-loss books. His mission is to guarantee weight loss for busy people. Science has proven that fitness begins in the kitchen, not in the gym. By merging breakthrough dietary science with great taste, he produces delicious belly-fat-melting menus.

Jorge has appeared on numerous television shows including the *Today* show, the *Dr. Oz Show,* the *Rachael Ray Show, Good Morning America, The View,* and *LIVE with Kelly and Michael.*

Follow Jorge at Facebook.com/JorgeCruiseFan, Twitter.com/JorgeCruise, Pinterest.com/JorgeCruise, YouTube.com/JorgeCruise, Instagram.com/Jorge Cruise, Plus.Google.com/JorgeCruise, and JorgeCruise.Tumblr.com.

FREE MENU
FOR WOMEN OVER 40

Go to JorgeCruise.com to get my FREE menu, as well as my report on the special dangers of sugar to women over 40. Included is the newest research on why weight loss on a biological level has been challenging in each age group and how men are affected as well.

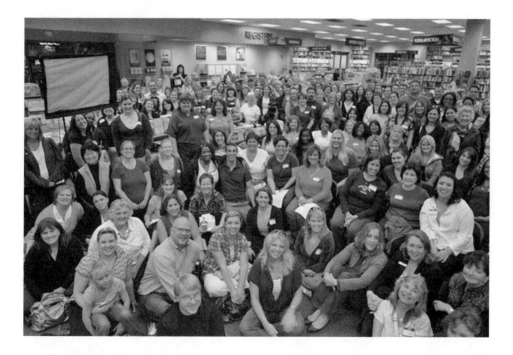

Visit JorgeCruise.com
and get the report for free!